CORNERSMITH
SALADS & PICKLES

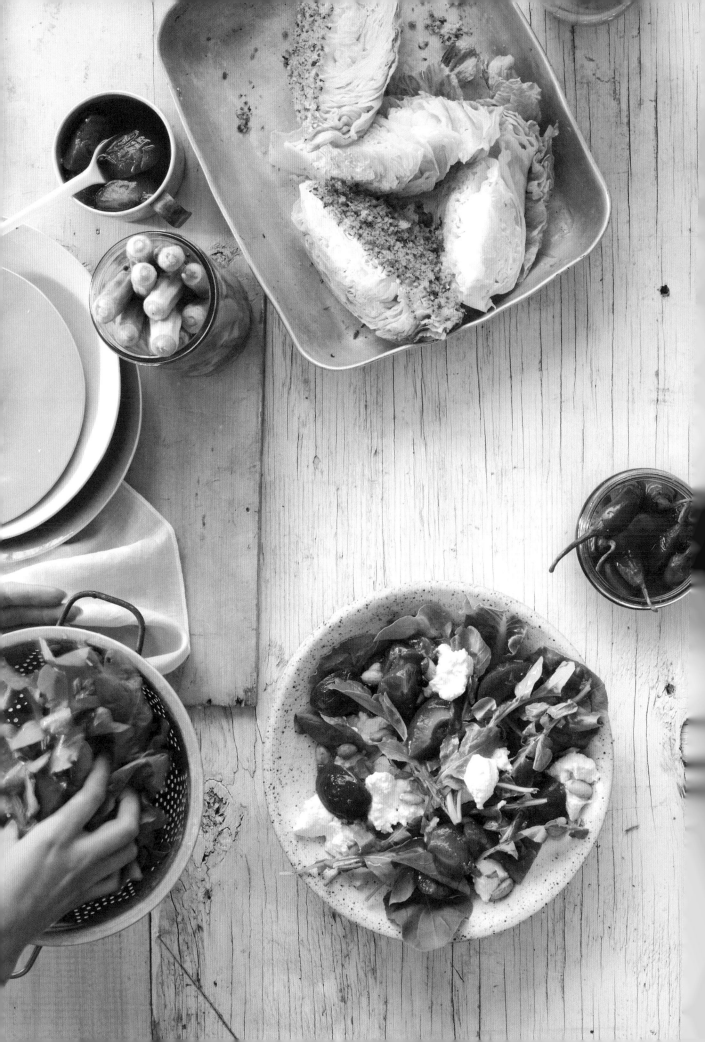

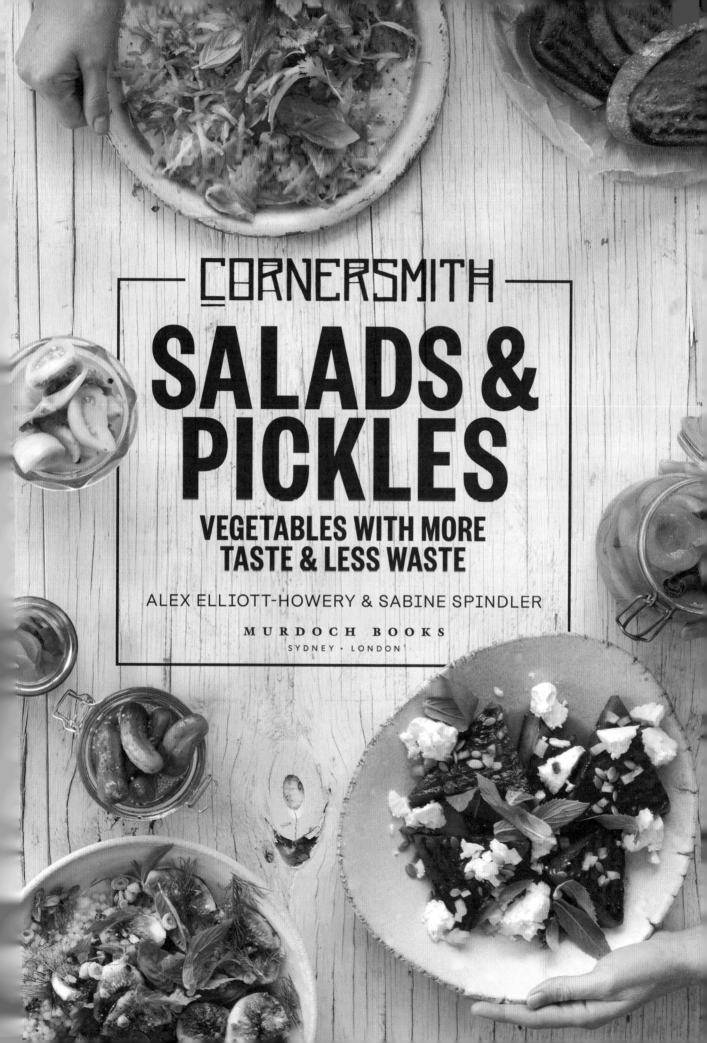

CORNERSMITH
SALADS & PICKLES
VEGETABLES WITH MORE TASTE & LESS WASTE

ALEX ELLIOTT-HOWERY & SABINE SPINDLER

MURDOCH BOOKS
SYDNEY · LONDON

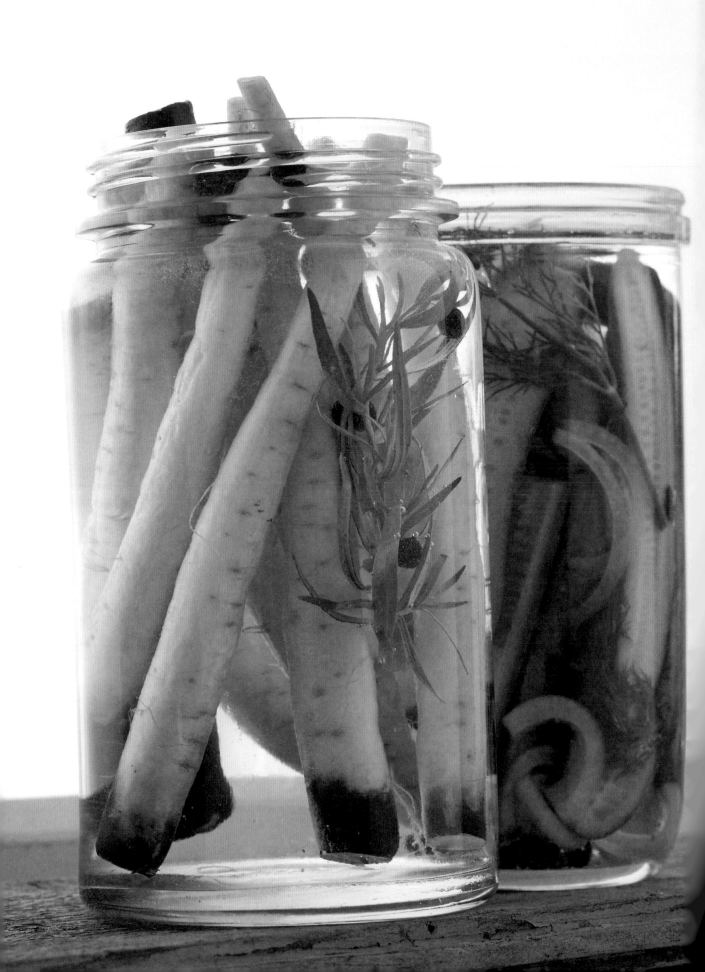

CONTENTS

INTRODUCTION

When we started out back in 2011, our neighbourhood cafe was a little shop with a big heart and a strong conscience when it came to sustainably sourced food. We could never have imagined how quickly Cornersmith would be embraced by the local community, and how so many customers would connect with what we were trying to do.

Cornersmith now consists of two cafes in Sydney – one in Marrickville and a newer venue in Annandale – as well as a Picklery, where we make our preserves, run our busy cooking school and sell preserving supplies. We have taught many hundreds of classes in pickling, fermenting, cheesemaking, bread baking and more over the years.

We think part of the reason Cornersmith has been embraced by so many is because we combine really delicious food with a solid commitment to good food choices. From the start we were determined that our food would be full of flavour, good for the person eating it and good for the planet. Nothing about this philosophy has changed as we've grown.

We only use seasonal produce; we support local small-scale producers who we admire; we're obsessive about preserving foods and reducing food waste; we only use small amounts of ethically raised meats and true free-range eggs; and we're committed to our community and food education.

But we don't expect people to love us unless the food tastes great. And it does – in no small part because of our brilliant head chef, Sabine Spindler, who shares our vision and beliefs and makes the best-tasting food we've ever eaten!

When I first met Sabine, I knew it would be an exciting food adventure if we put our heads together. We come from very different backgrounds, but we have a shared obsession with delicious food, food education and reducing food waste.

I had spent the previous 10 years cooking for my family, devouring wholefoods cookbooks and reading everything I could get my hands on about the issues in our current food system. I decided to teach myself how to cook everything from scratch as a way of being less reliant on supermarkets and more connected to what I was buying and feeding my young family.

I became interested in ways to reduce food waste on a domestic level, teaching myself how to preserve as a way of dealing with excess fruit and vegetables. I bottled home-grown vegetables, made jams from neighbours' unloved fruit trees, and pickled what was left over in the fridge at the end of the week.

Sabine had trained as a chef in her home country Germany, and worked in fine-dining restaurants all over Europe. The food she learnt to cook was always focused on seasonal produce, which gave her an early appreciation of the work that farmers, producers and growers do. But she was shocked by how much food was wasted on a daily basis in these top restaurants. Chefs have the skills to make use of every part of the plant or the animal, but were still encouraged to throw out large quantities of perfectly good produce.

Sabine grew up with two grandmothers who had lived through wartime rationing, when preserving and avoiding waste was a matter of survival. They impressed upon her the importance of using everything you have and not wasting a morsel.

This book is an extension of our shared love of vegetables, as well as a bit of a roadmap for where we think the future of food needs to head — more vegetables, less meat; more cooking from scratch; less waste, more preserving; more sharing and community building.

We've chosen to make a cookbook about salads and pickles because we think it best represents the way we eat, and because these are the two reasons people keep coming back to eat with us. We're known for our love of vegetables and the way we make them taste so good — so good, in fact, that they're the hero on our plates.

We want to encourage people to really understand the seasons, and we hope this book helps you to navigate seasonal eating; we want you to think about where your produce is coming from and who you're supporting when you purchase your groceries.

We want you to question what a meal needs to look like. The way we eat at Cornersmith is about assembling a variety of delicious elements. We make one or two interesting vegetable dishes, open a jar of pickles or ferments, add a nice loaf of bread and then a small simple protein — a lovely piece of cheese, some boiled eggs, a grilled piece of fish or meat.

While a lot of thought and planning goes into our menus, we are not interested in tricked-up faddy food — no diets, no superfoods, no guilt. Cornersmith is about simple, tasty meals, made from scratch with care.

Pickling and preserving is what we're known for. We pickle not just because we love the taste, but because pickling is an important food tradition that needs to be understood and passed down the generations. Preserving makes you understand the seasons, helps you to know what's going into your food, and avoid unnecessary preservatives and packaging. It also massively reduces food waste. On top of all of that it's good fun!

Having a pantry full of pickles very quickly makes a meal more interesting. If you can toss some sliced pickled ginger through a noodle dish or throw some pickled peaches through a leafy green salad, you'll not only have something incredibly delicious, but you'll know you preserved the best of the season to use any time of the year. A home-made relish will make your work sandwiches a whole lot more exciting, and you'll be the hero of the barbecue if you bring a few jars of delicious chutney.

Not only is this book full of our favourite seasonal recipes, we've included tips on growing your own sprouts at home (see page 130), and even flavouring your own salts (page 72) and vinegars (page 164).

At the back of this book you'll find Sabine's guide on how to make the best salad dressings using what's in your fridge and pantry (page 205), and an introduction to pickling (page 209) and fermenting (page 216), to keep your preserving worries at bay!

One of the most important elements of what we do at Cornersmith and what this book is about is getting people to rethink their kitchen food waste at home. This book is full of tips and quick tricks for using up what's left in the fridge at the end of the week; our recipes and ideas will show you how to use that little bit of ginger left over, the tops of your leeks, your parsley stems, and even your pineapple skins!

These are all little things that can make a big difference in reducing the amount that ends up in your bin, as well as to your household budget.

We are incredibly lucky that all the 'Smithies' who work with us are as committed to reducing food waste as we are. Throughout our shops, there are chefs, picklers and baristas constantly coming up with innovative ways to make sure nothing goes in the bin or down the sink that doesn't absolutely have to.

Recently we've rescued 130 kg (nearly 300 lb) of organic strawberries that would have ended up in landfill simply because they didn't meet supermarket-shelving standards. We turned eight boxes of mushrooms left over from a photo shoot into dehydrated mushies for winter broths. So stay tuned, because we're only getting stronger and bolder with our long-term war on food waste.

Alex Elliott-Howery

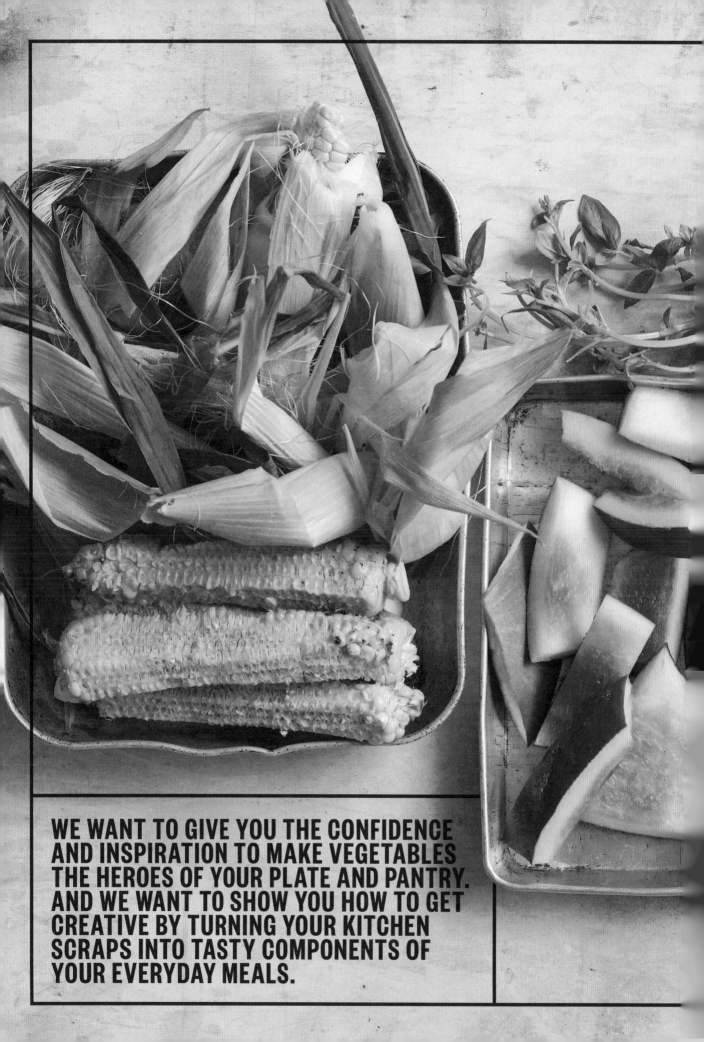

WE WANT TO GIVE YOU THE CONFIDENCE AND INSPIRATION TO MAKE VEGETABLES THE HEROES OF YOUR PLATE AND PANTRY. AND WE WANT TO SHOW YOU HOW TO GET CREATIVE BY TURNING YOUR KITCHEN SCRAPS INTO TASTY COMPONENTS OF YOUR EVERYDAY MEALS.

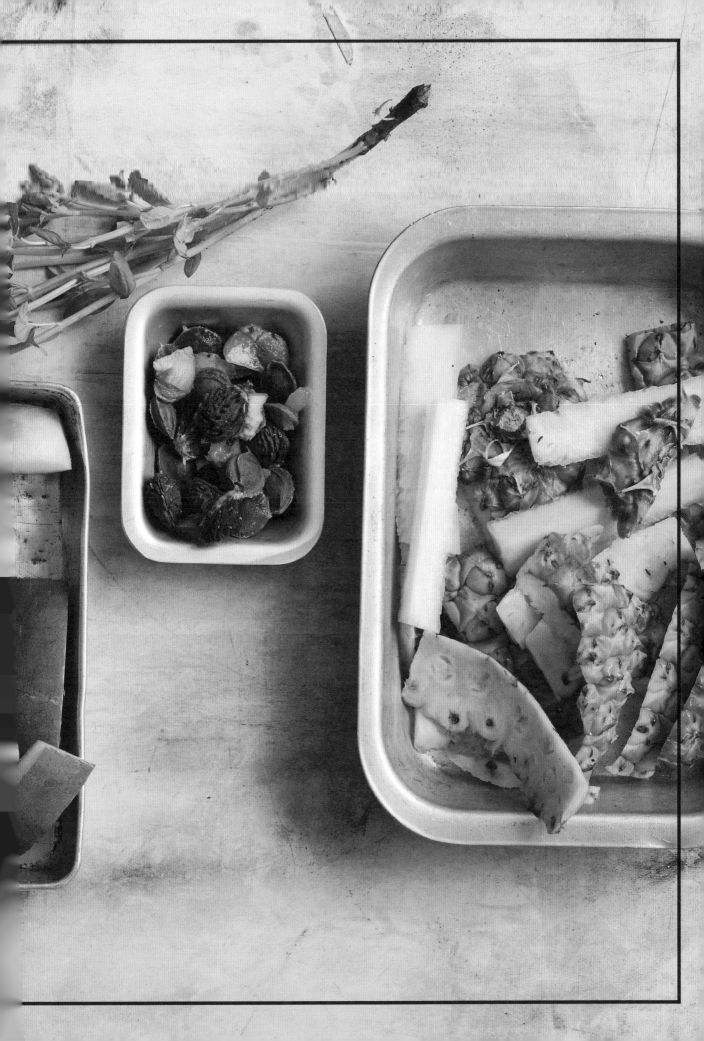

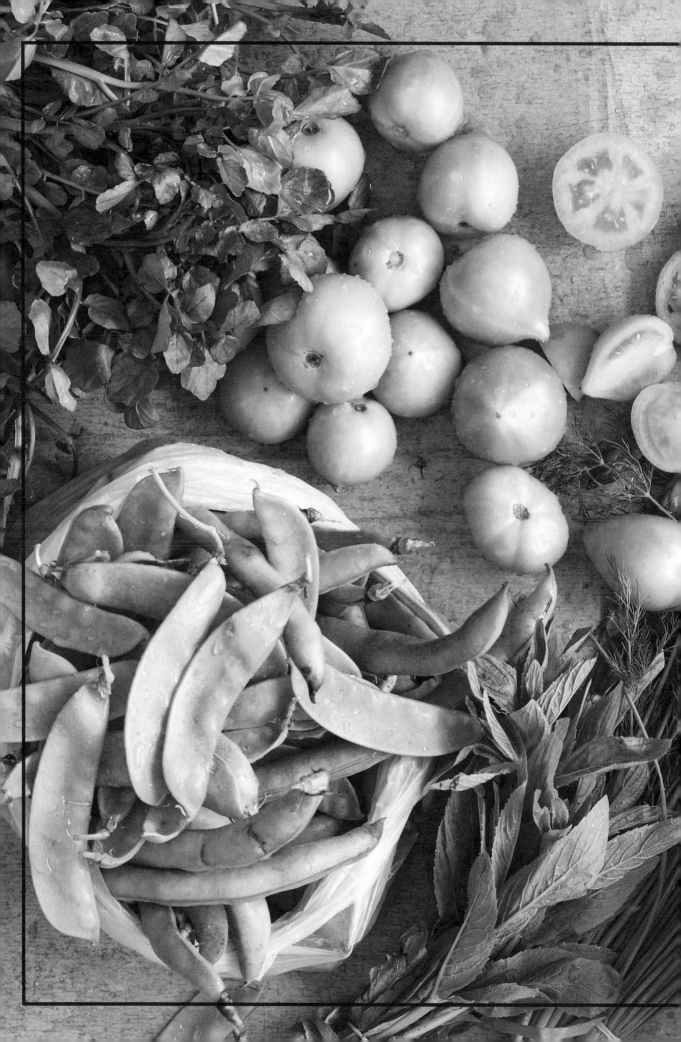

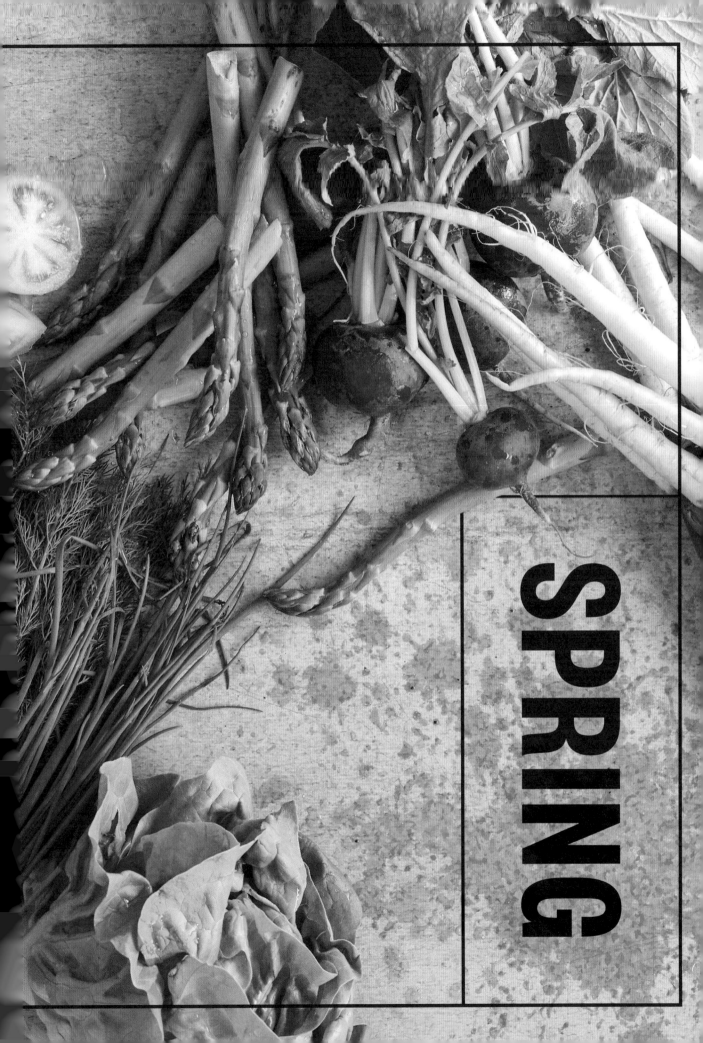

SPRING

PREPARATION TIME	COOKING TIME	SERVES
25 minutes, plus overnight soaking	25 minutes	4

When it's broad bean and pea season, you should eat them every day! This salad stars freekeh, a delicious, highly nutritious grain made from roasted green (early harvest) wheat. If you can't obtain it, use barley, spelt or other grains instead.

This salad looks great on a large flat platter. You could also double the quantity and take it to a barbecue or picnic.

BROAD BEAN & PEA SALAD WITH FREEKEH & YOGHURT SAUCE

160 g (5½ oz/¾ cup) freekeh, soaked overnight
125 g (4½ oz) podded fresh peas
350 g (12 oz) podded fresh broad beans
60 ml (2 fl oz/¼ cup) olive oil, plus extra for drizzling over the salad
1 large brown onion, thinly sliced
1½ tablespoons chopped dill, including the stems
juice of ½–1 lemon, to taste
⅓ cup picked dill and mint leaves, torn just before serving
ground sumac, for sprinkling (optional)

YOGHURT SAUCE
200 g (7 oz/¾ cup) natural unsweetened yoghurt
2 garlic cloves, crushed
pinch of salt
pinch of chilli powder or cayenne pepper

Bring a saucepan of salted water to the boil. Drain and rinse the freekeh, add it to the pan and cook for 6–8 minutes, or until the grains are just tender, but still retain their shape. Drain and set aside to cool.

Meanwhile, bring another saucepan of water to the boil. Blanch the peas for 1 minute, then remove with a slotted spoon. Refresh them under cold water, drain well and set aside.

Bring the water back to the boil and blanch the broad beans for about 2 minutes. Drain, then refresh under cold water. When cool enough to handle, peel off and discard the outer skin. Set the broad beans aside, keeping them separate to the peas.

Combine the yoghurt sauce ingredients in a bowl, mixing until smooth. Set aside.

Pour the olive oil into a frying pan large enough to hold the broad beans in one flat layer. Heat over medium–high heat. Add the onion, season with salt and pepper, then let it soften over medium–low heat for 5–10 minutes, stirring now and then.

Turn the heat back up to high. Add the broad beans and stir-fry for 2–4 minutes, or until they turn golden brown. Add the chopped dill and turn off the heat.

In a mixing bowl, combine the fried broad beans and peas. Season with salt, pepper and lemon juice to taste.

To serve, spread the cooked freekeh on a platter, arrange the broad beans and peas on top and drizzle with the yoghurt sauce. Finish with the torn dill and mint, a sprinkling of sumac, if desired, and an extra drizzle of olive oil.

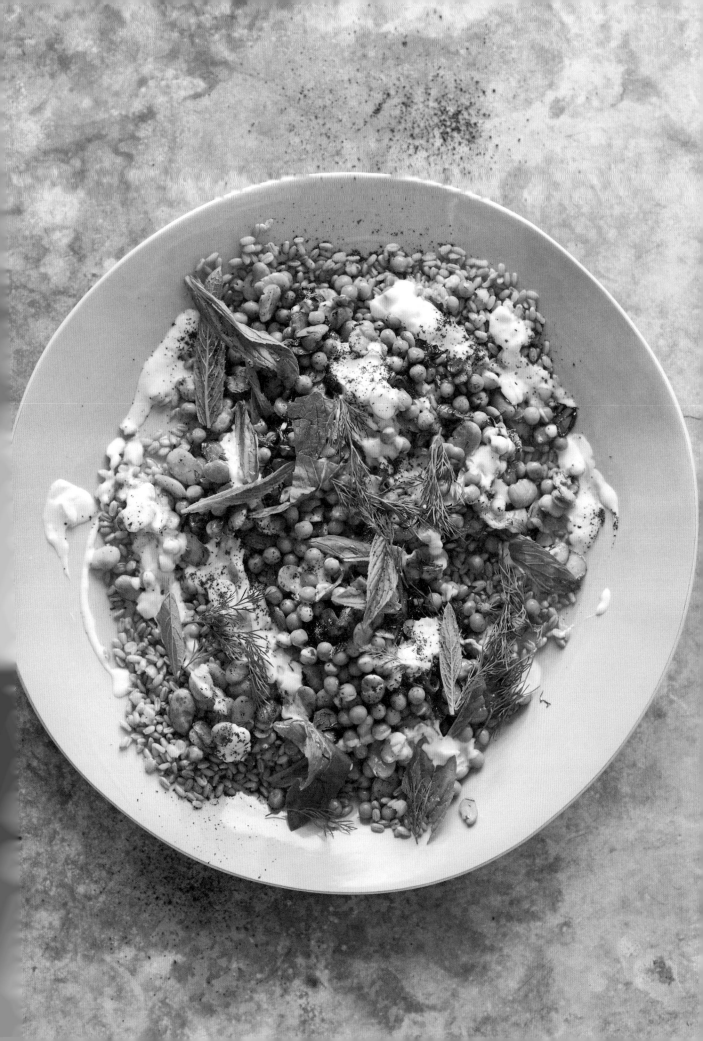

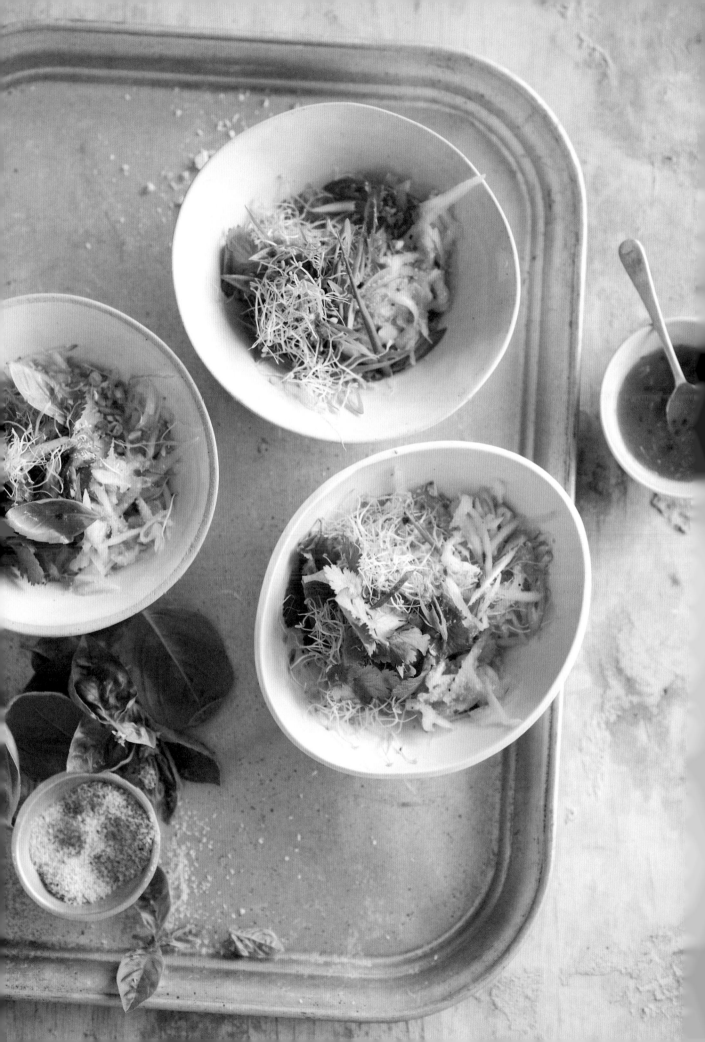

PREPARATION TIME	COOKING TIME	SERVES
20 minutes	5 minutes	4

This is our version of a very delicious salad from South-East Asia. We make it using our Lime Pickle (page 134) and Lime Vinegar (page 167), and sometimes add our Turmeric Pickled Mango (page 42) as well. These are all handy condiments to have in the cupboard, but if you don't, you can use a good lime pickle from an Indian grocery store, and make a quick lime vinegar using equal quantities of lime juice and white wine vinegar.

You could experiment by adding a splash of fish or soy sauce as well.

GREEN MANGO & PAPAYA SALAD

Place the coconut in a dry frying pan over medium–low heat. Toast the coconut without any oil, stirring all the time, for 2–3 minutes, or until it turns golden. Tip into a small bowl and set aside.

Mix all the dressing ingredients in a bowl until the sugar and salt have dissolved. The dressing should be a subtle balance of sweet, sour, spicy and salty, so adjust the flavour to your liking.

Peel the mangoes and papaya, and remove the seeds from the papaya. Grate the mangoes and papaya coarsely into a mixing bowl, avoiding the flat stone in the middle of the mangoes.

Add the sprouts, coriander, spring onion and half the toasted coconut, then add the dressing and toss together gently. Check the seasoning again.

Place the salad on a serving platter or in a bowl. Sprinkle with the cashews, basil and remaining coconut and serve.

25 g (1 oz/¼ cup) desiccated (shredded) coconut
2 green unripe mangoes
250–300 g (9–10½ oz) green papaya
60 g (2¼ oz/1 cup) alfalfa or lentil sprouts (to grow your own, see page 130)
1 large handful of picked coriander (cilantro) leaves
4 spring onions (scallions), thinly sliced on a slight angle
40 g (1½ oz/¼ cup) toasted cashews (see page 206), finely chopped
1 large handful of picked basil leaves

LIME DRESSING
60 ml (2 fl oz/¼ cup) lime juice
2 tablespoons Lime Vinegar (page 167)
2 teaspoons Lime Pickle (page 134), finely chopped into a smooth purée
¼ teaspoon chilli flakes
pinch of cayenne pepper
2½ teaspoons brown or raw sugar
2 teaspoons salt

PREPARATION TIME	COOKING TIME	SERVES
20 minutes	10 minutes	4

Kohlrabi is part of the cabbage family. A long over-looked vegetable, we're pleased to see it finding its way back into kitchens. Its flavour is a bit sweeter than regular cabbage, which works really well in this salad with the sharpness of the radish. Charring it on the barbecue brings out its sweetness even more.

KOHLRABI, RADISH & TOFU WITH MISO DRESSING

1 small green or purple kohlrabi, about 200 g (7 oz)
4 small radishes, tender leaves intact
2 medium–large radishes
2 teaspoons vegetable oil
2 young small bok choy (pak choy)
2 teaspoons lemon juice
300 g (10½ oz) firm tofu, cut into bite-sized cubes
1 tablespoon finely snipped chives

MISO DRESSING
1 tablespoon Ginger-Infused Vinegar (page 167; see tip)
½ teaspoon chopped infused ginger (from the Ginger-Infused Vinegar; see tip)
1½ teaspoons miso paste
1 teaspoon tahini
½ teaspoon hot water
¼ teaspoon sugar
pinch of salt
1 tablespoon olive oil

To make the dressing, whisk all the ingredients except the olive oil in a bowl until smooth, then slowly whisk in the olive oil. Set aside.

Heat a barbecue or chargrill pan to medium–high.

Meanwhile, peel the kohlrabi, trim off the top and bottom, then cut it in half. Set one half aside.

Cut the other kohlrabi half into segments about 3–5 mm (⅛–¼ inch) thick and place in a mixing bowl. Wash and dry all the radishes. Pick the leaves from the small radishes and add them to the kohlrabi segments. Cut the small radishes in half and add them to the bowl as well. Sprinkle with the vegetable oil, season with salt and gently mix together.

Char the kohlrabi segments and radish halves on the hot barbecue or chargrill pan for 2–3 minutes, turning them over halfway through. Remove from the heat.

Thinly slice the reserved kohlrabi half and the larger radishes using a mandoline. Place in a mixing bowl.

Wash and dry the bok choy, cut lengthways into quarters and add to the bowl, along with the charred vegetables. Sprinkle with the lemon juice and season with salt and pepper. Carefully mix the tofu through.

Arrange the salad in a large bowl or on a platter. Drizzle with the miso dressing, garnish with the chives and serve.

TIP: If you don't have any Ginger-Infused Vinegar and infused ginger, grate 1 tablespoon fresh ginger into 3 tablespoons apple cider vinegar or white wine vinegar and leave to infuse for 10–15 minutes before using.

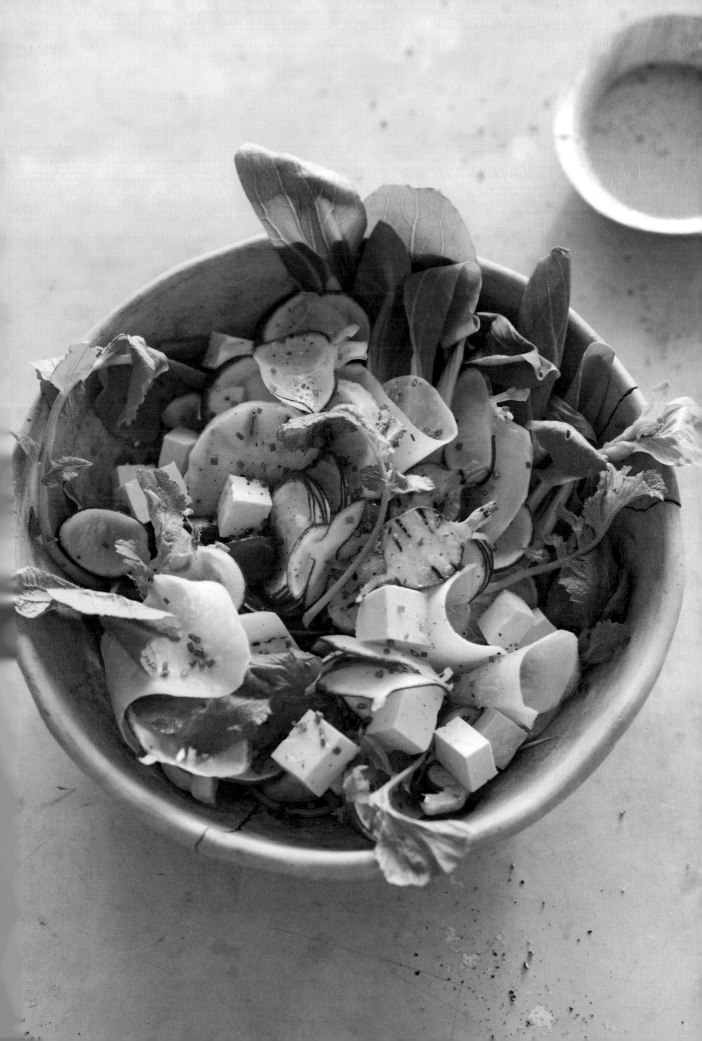

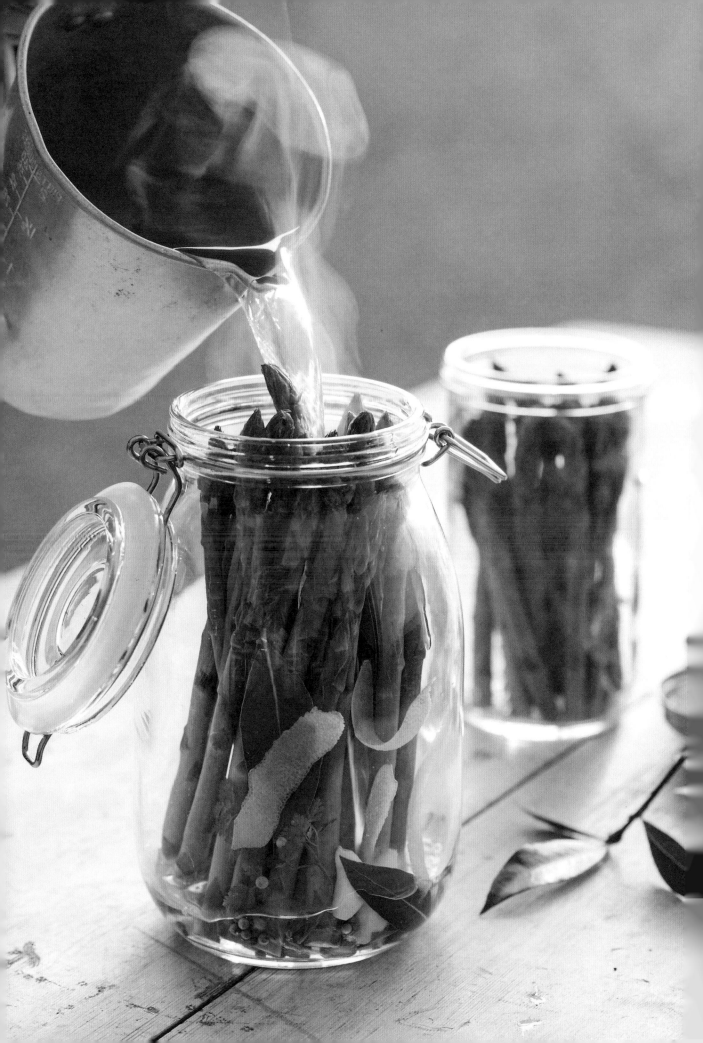

PREPARATION TIME	STORAGE	MAKES
20 minutes, plus 20 minutes sterilising	3 months in the pantry, or 6 months in the fridge	2 x 500 ml (17 fl oz/2 cup) jars

We like to make these pickles all through asparagus season in spring. They're great thinly sliced through salads, on an antipasto plate, or just straight out of the jar. Storing them in the fridge, rather than the cupboard, helps the asparagus retain its colour and crunch.

PICKLED ASPARAGUS WITH GARLIC & LEMON

Sterilise your jars and lids (see page 212).

Meanwhile, make your brine by combining the vinegar, sugar, salt and water in a non-reactive, medium-sized saucepan. Place over low heat and stir to dissolve the sugar and salt. Add the thyme sprigs, bay leaves, garlic cloves, lemon peel strips and peppercorns and slowly bring to simmering point.

Wash and dry your asparagus. If the spears are very long, cut them in half.

When the jars are cool enough to handle, use a clean pair of tongs to add 4 lemon peel strips from the brine to each jar, along with 2 garlic cloves, 2 thyme sprigs, 2 bay leaves and ½ teaspoon peppercorns. Now carefully pack the raw asparagus in — you should be able to get about 10 spears into each jar.

Cover the asparagus with the hot brine, making sure the asparagus is completely submerged under the vinegar. Tuck the asparagus stems down under the shoulders of the jars if you need to.

Remove any air bubbles by gently tapping each jar on the work surface and sliding a clean butter knife or chopstick around the inside to release any hidden air pockets. Wipe the rims of the jars with paper towel or a clean damp cloth and seal immediately.

You can store these pickles in the cupboard for up to 3 months. We prefer to keep them in the fridge, as the cold helps the asparagus spears keep their crunch; they will last in the fridge for up to 6 months. Try to let them sit for 2–4 weeks before eating.

375 ml (13 fl oz/1½ cups) white wine vinegar
75 g (2½ oz/⅓ cup) sugar
1½ teaspoons salt
375 ml (13 fl oz/1½ cups) water
4 thyme sprigs
4 bay leaves
4 garlic cloves, peeled
8 strips of lemon peel
1 teaspoon white peppercorns
about 20 asparagus spears

TIP: This is a good recipe for pickling any woody stems you have trimmed off asparagus while preparing the spears for steaming. Peel those woody end bits and cover them with this brine instead of tossing them in the bin or compost heap. Then toss them through a green salad!

PREPARATION TIME	HEAT-PROCESSING	STORAGE	MAKES
20 minutes, plus 1 hour salting, plus 20 minutes sterilising	15 minutes	up to 2 years	3–4 × 500 ml (17 fl oz/2 cup) jars

Green tomatoes — unripe red tomatoes — are our favourite spring vegetable. Tart, crunchy and delicious, they make the best pickles, and these ones just get better and better with time.

Ask your local greengrocer to get you a box of green tomatoes, so you can make a big batch of these pickles. Your friends and neighbours will love it when you share these around.

PICKLED GREEN TOMATOES

1 kg (2 lb 4 oz) green tomatoes
1 large onion, thinly sliced
    (optional)
1 tablespoon salt
750 ml (26 fl oz/3 cups)
    white wine vinegar
375 ml (13 fl oz/1½ cups) water
165 g (5¾ oz/¾ cup) sugar
½ teaspoon ground turmeric
3–4 cinnamon sticks
6–8 garlic cloves, peeled
3–4 strips of lemon peel
3–4 bay leaves
1½–2 teaspoons black
    peppercorns

First, prepare your tomatoes. Cut any larger tomatoes into quarters or thick slices, and smaller tomatoes in half. Place in a large bowl. Mix the onion through, if using, then sprinkle with the salt. Allow to sit for 2 hours, or even overnight, to draw the excess moisture out.

Make your brine by combining the vinegar, water, sugar and turmeric in a non-reactive, medium-sized saucepan over low heat. Stir to dissolve the sugar, then bring to simmering point.

Meanwhile, sterilise your jars and lids (see page 212).

When the jars are cool enough to handle, drain off and discard the excess liquid from your tomatoes. To each jar, add 1 cinnamon stick, 2 garlic cloves, a lemon peel strip, a bay leaf and ½ teaspoon peppercorns. Using small clean tongs or clean hands, carefully but tightly pack the tomato pieces into the jars. Pour the hot brine over until the tomatoes are completely covered.

Remove any air bubbles by gently tapping each jar on the work surface and sliding a clean butter knife or chopstick around the inside to release any hidden air pockets. Wipe the rims of the jars with paper towel or a clean damp cloth and seal immediately.

Heat-process (see page 211) for 15 minutes, then allow to cool.

These pickles will keep in a cool, dark place for up to 2 years, but do let them sit for at least 1 month before you try them; they'll be even better after 3 months. Once opened, refrigerate and use within 6 months.

TIP: The garlic cloves will take on a blue/grey hue with time, in reaction to the vinegar. Blanching them in boiling water for 10 seconds before adding them to the pickling jars will stop any discolouration.

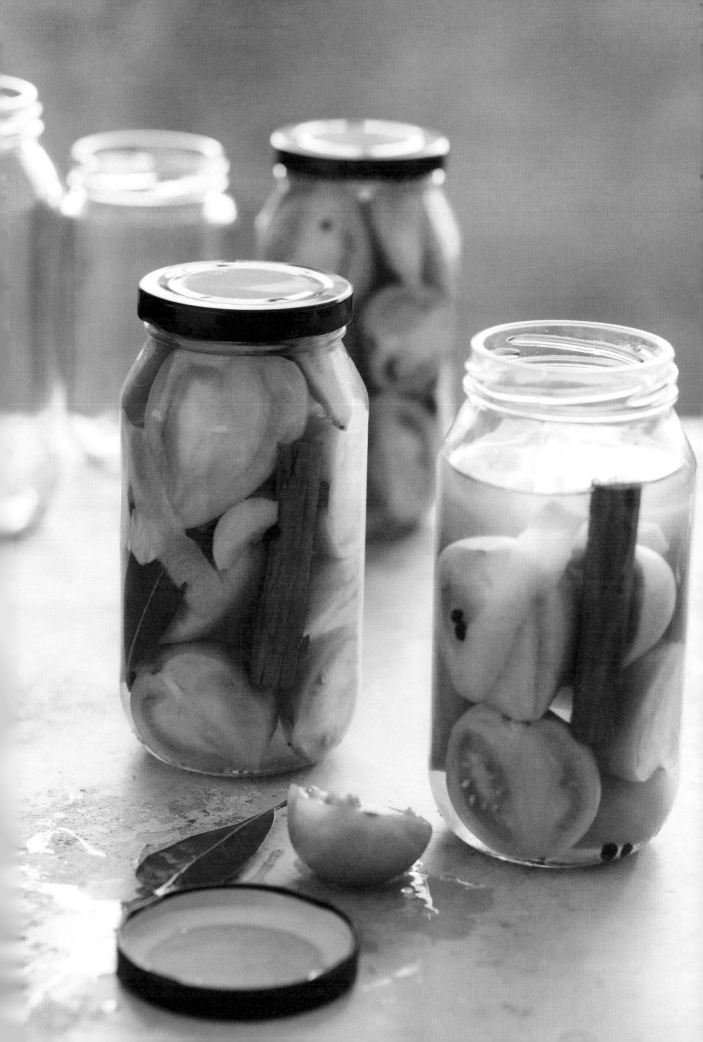

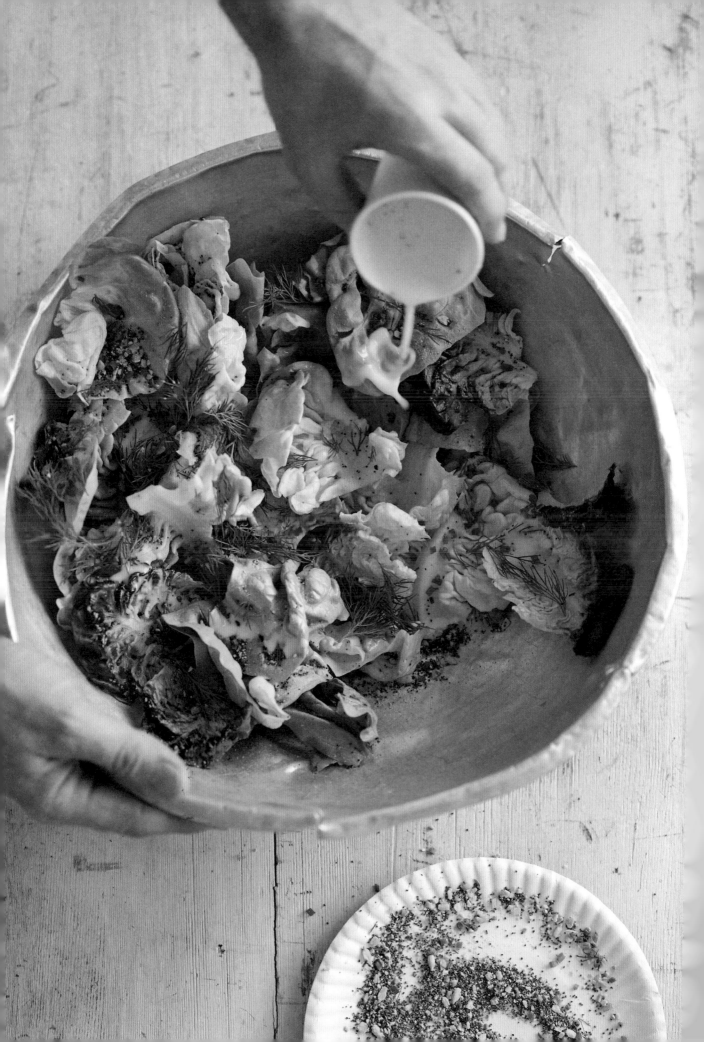

PREPARATION TIME	COOKING TIME	SERVES
15 minutes	about 5 minutes	4

A beautiful addition to any meal, this simple leafy salad stands out because of the sweetness of the dressing, and the texture of the poppy and sunflower seeds. You could also use goat's milk yoghurt or regular cow's milk yoghurt in the dressing.

LEAFY SALAD WITH POPPY SEEDS & SHEEP'S MILK YOGHURT DRESSING

In a dry frying pan, lightly toast the poppy seeds over medium heat, without any oil, for 2–3 minutes, tossing frequently so they don't burn. Tip the seeds into a mortar and set aside.

In the same pan, toast the sunflower seeds until lightly browned, then tip them onto a chopping board and roughly chop. Add them to the poppy seeds and grind into a coarse 'dust' using a pestle. Set aside.

Discard the outer leaves from the lettuces. Tear the inner leaves into bite-sized pieces and place in a large mixing bowl.

To prepare the dressing, combine the lemon juice, honey and yoghurt in a small bowl. Season with salt and pepper and whisk until smooth. You want a balance between acidity and sweetness, so add more lemon juice or honey if necessary.

Pour the yoghurt dressing over the lettuce leaves, add half the dill and chives and gently toss to combine.

Place the salad in a serving bowl. Sprinkle with the poppy seed 'dust' and remaining dill and chives.

Serve immediately.

1½ teaspoons poppy seeds
1 tablespoon sunflower seeds
½ baby cos (romaine) lettuce
½ butter lettuce
½ cup picked dill
2 tablespoons finely snipped chives

SHEEP'S MILK YOGHURT DRESSING
juice of ½ lemon
1½ teaspoons runny honey
2 tablespoons sheep's milk yoghurt

PREPARATION TIME	COOKING TIME	SERVES
25 minutes (including 15 minutes soaking)	25 minutes	4

This is a very Italian way to prepare zucchini, almost like an antipasti. Pan-fried, then gently braised, the zucchini tastes so good with fennel seeds, garlic, chilli and lemon zest — with sultanas adding a hint of sweetness. We decided to turn this dish into a warm salad, to really let the flavours sing.

WARM ZUCCHINI SALAD

1½ tablespoons olive oil, plus extra for drizzling over the salad
6 small or 5 medium-sized zucchini (courgettes), about 550–600 g (1 lb 4 oz–1 lb 5 oz), sliced about 2 cm (¾ inch) thick
1 garlic clove, crushed
¼ teaspoon fennel seeds
2 pinches of chilli flakes
zest and juice of ½ lemon
2–3 thyme sprigs
a pinch of salt
1 tablespoon sultanas (golden raisins)
3 cups picked parsley leaves
1 tablespoon chopped tarragon
80–100 g (2¾ oz–3½ oz) fresh ricotta cheese

Add the olive oil to a saucepan large enough to fit all the zucchini slices in one layer. Heat over medium–high heat, then add the zucchini slices, in one flat layer. Cook for 5–6 minutes, or until golden brown.

Flip the zucchini slices over. Sprinkle with the garlic, fennel seeds, chilli flakes, lemon zest, thyme sprigs and salt. Put the lid on, reduce the heat to very low and let the zucchini cook for 10–15 minutes, until turning soft.

Turn off the heat and let the zucchini sit in the pan, with the lid on, for another 5–10 minutes.

Meanwhile, soak the sultanas in a little hot water for 10–15 minutes, then drain and finely chop. Set aside.

Place the warm zucchini slices in a large mixing bowl and 'tear' them apart with the side of a spoon. Add the chopped sultanas, parsley, tarragon and lemon juice and mix together gently.

Place the salad in a serving dish. Finish with dollops of the ricotta and an extra drizzle of olive oil. Grind some black pepper over the top and serve immediately.

TIP: Cook the zucchini a little bit longer with the lid on, then mash it with a fork and serve as a delicious dip for scooping up with crusty sourdough, or tossed through hot pasta.

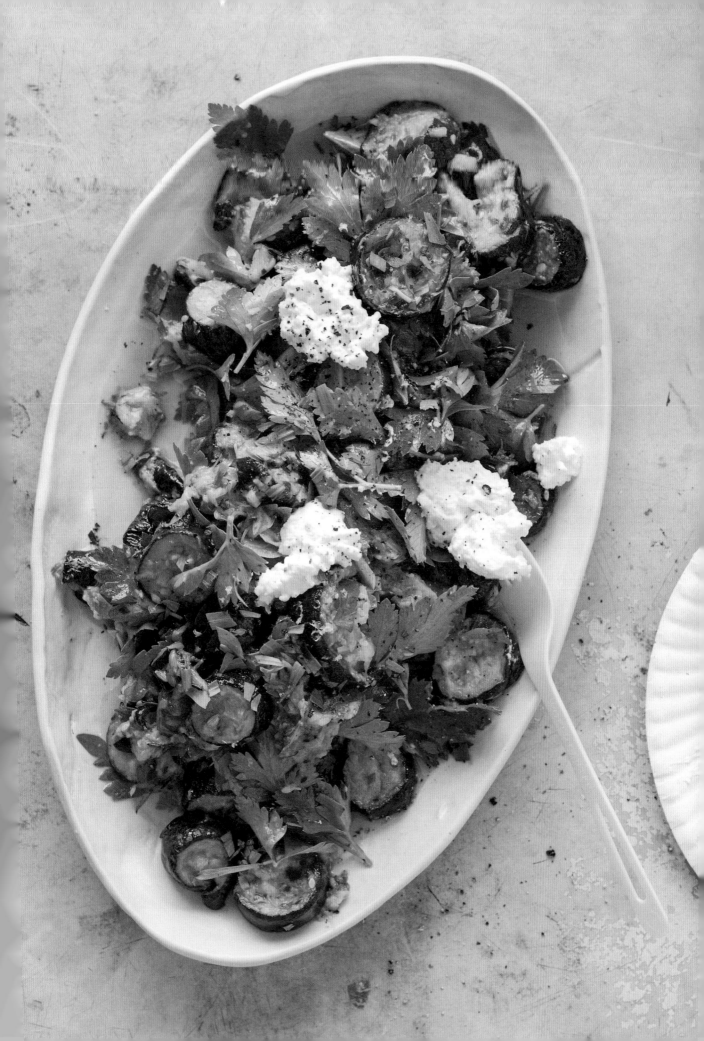

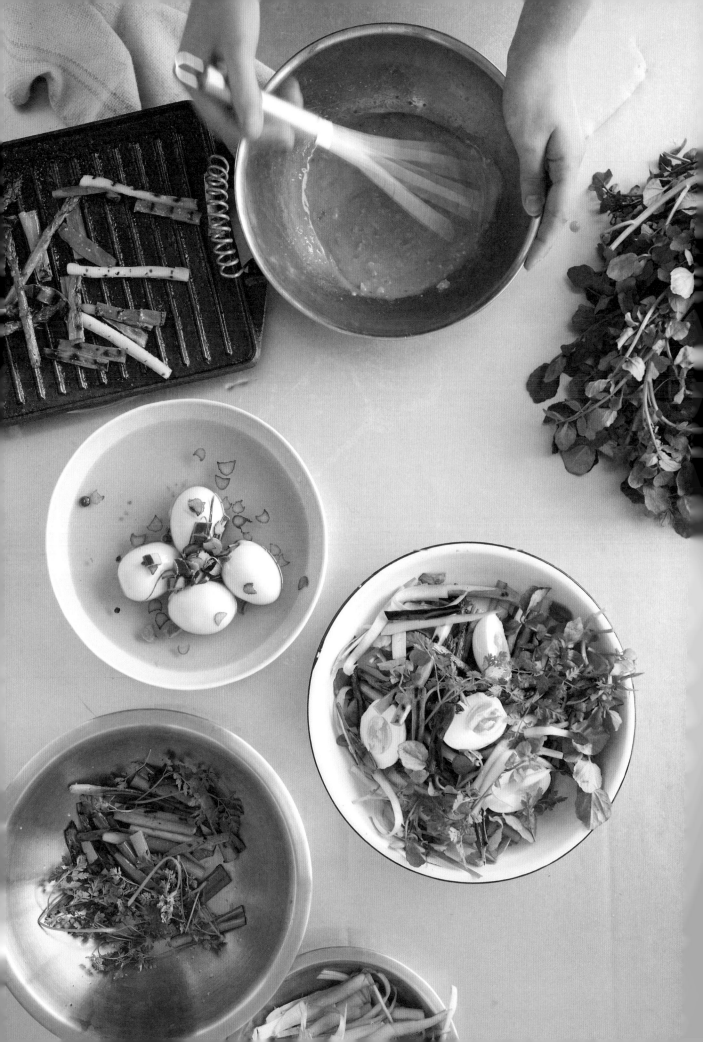

PREPARATION TIME	COOKING TIME	SERVES
15 minutes	10 minutes	4

Very pretty and green, this salad makes a lovely lunch in spring. It's also a great use for the Pink Pickled Eggs on page 28. If you don't have any handy, serve the salad with soft-boiled or poached eggs instead.

ASPARAGUS & WATERCRESS WITH WALNUT & ORANGE VINAIGRETTE

Heat a barbecue or chargrill pan to medium–high.

Meanwhile, trim the woody ends from the asparagus and reserve them for quick pickling (see page 162). Cut the top of the asparagus spears into 10 cm (4 inch) lengths and place in a mixing bowl. Slice the remaining asparagus pieces lengthways using a mandoline, then set aside, keeping them separate.

Trim the spring onions. Cut the white ends into 12 cm (4½ inch) lengths and add them to the mixing bowl. Cut the remaining green bits into 6 cm (2½ inch) lengths and set aside, keeping them separate.

Season the vegetables in the bowl with salt and pepper. Add the olive oil and gently mix until well coated with the oil, then place them on the hot barbecue or chargrill pan. Cook the spring onions for 3–5 minutes, and the asparagus tips for about 5–6 minutes, or until charred on the outside and still a bit crunchy inside. Then add the spring onion greens and quickly char them for 1 minute. Place the cooked vegetables into a large mixing bowl and let them cool down.

Meanwhile, prepare the dressing. In a small bowl, combine the vinegar, anchovies and mustard. Season with salt and pepper, then whisk in the olive oil in a slow stream. Add the chopped walnuts.

To the bowl of charred vegetables, add the raw asparagus slices, watercress and half the chervil, mixing gently. Add the walnut dressing and toss gently.

Place the salad in a serving bowl, garnish with the remaining chervil and the pickled eggs and serve.

12 asparagus spears
6 small spring onions (scallions)
1½ teaspoons olive oil
2 large handfuls of picked watercress
1 small handful of picked chervil leaves
2 Pink Pickled Eggs (page 28), cut in half or quarters lengthways

WALNUT & ORANGE VINAIGRETTE
3 teaspoons Orange Vinegar (page 167), or apple cider vinegar mixed with a squeeze of orange juice
2 anchovy fillets, rinsed and finely chopped
1 teaspoon dijon mustard
80 ml (2½ fl oz/⅓ cup) olive oil
30 g (1 oz/¼ cup) walnuts, finely chopped

PREPARATION TIME	COOKING TIME	STORAGE	MAKES
15 minutes	about 15 minutes	up to 3 weeks	1 x 500 ml (17 fl oz/2 cup) jar

In this recipe you can also use the brine from another pickle to lightly pickle your eggs. We suggest the brine from the Pickled Rhubarb on page 31, as it gives the eggs a nice dusty pink colour; you could also use the brine from the Sweet Pickled Pears (page 200) or Malt Pickled Onions (page 161), or experiment with any other brines you have in the fridge. You'll need about 250 ml (9 fl oz/1 cup) of brine for a 500 ml (17 fl oz/2 cup) jar.

PINK PICKLED EGGS

5 free-range eggs
125 ml (4 fl oz/½ cup) red wine
    vinegar
140 g (5 oz/⅔ cup) raw sugar
60 ml (2 fl oz/¼ cup) water
2 teaspoons honey
10 g (¼ oz) knob of fresh ginger,
    washed but not peeled,
    cut into slices about 1 cm
    (½ inch) thick
4 allspice berries
4 black peppercorns
2 strips of orange peel

Because this recipe stays in the fridge, it doesn't need a sterilised jar, just a clean dry jar and lid.

Boil the eggs in a saucepan of water for 9 minutes; they need to be hard-boiled. Run the eggs under cool water, then carefully peel them. Place in a bowl and keep in the fridge until completely cool.

Meanwhile, make your brine by combining the vinegar, sugar, water and honey in a non-reactive, medium-sized saucepan. Place over low heat and stir to dissolve the sugar and honey. Add the spices and orange peel strips and slowly bring to simmering point. Turn off the heat and let the vinegar cool and flavours develop.

Once the eggs and the vinegar are cool, carefully pack the eggs into a clean jar, being careful not to break the whites. Pour the brine into the jar, making sure the eggs are completely submerged under the vinegar. Remove any air bubbles by gently tapping the jar on the work surface and sliding a clean butter knife or chopstick around the inside to release any hidden air pockets. Wipe the rim of the jar with paper towel or a clean damp cloth and seal.

Leave to sit in the fridge for at least 1 week before eating. The eggs will last for up to 3 weeks in the fridge, before they start to go a bit rubbery.

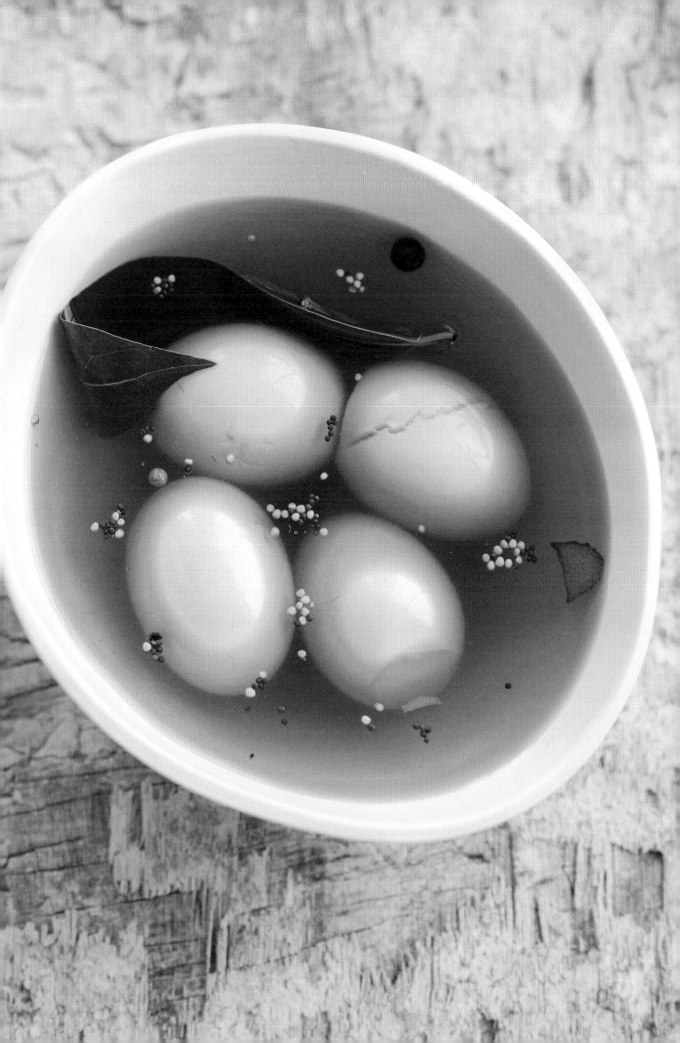

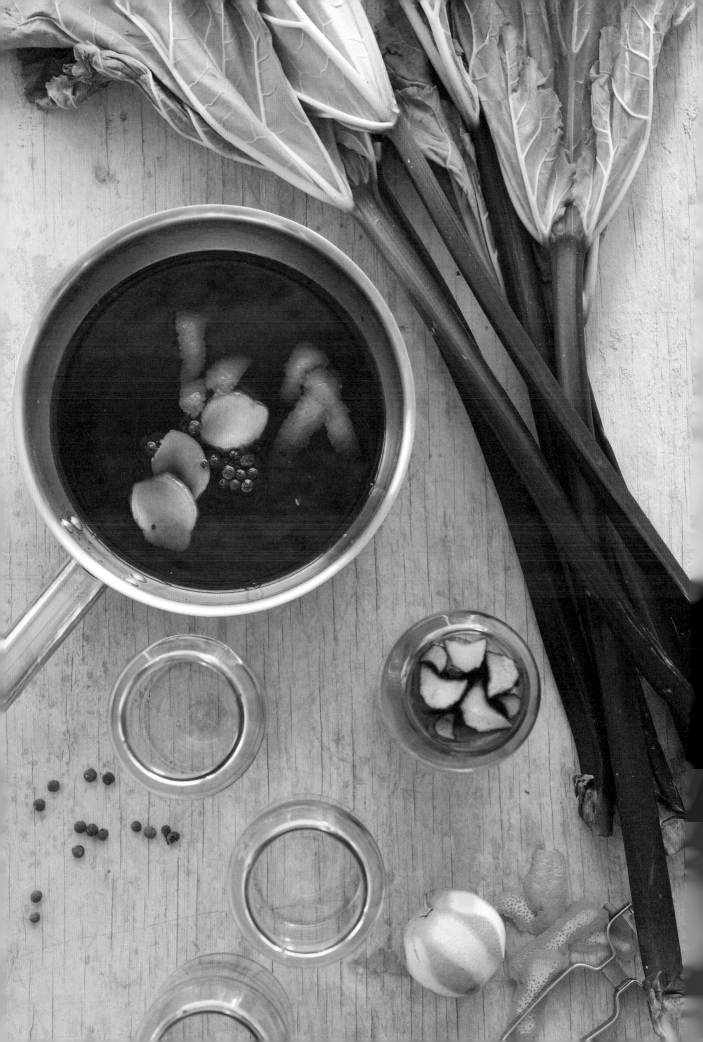

PREPARATION TIME	STORAGE	MAKES
20 minutes, plus 20 minutes sterilising, plus 10 minutes heat-prooooing (optional)	2–3 months, or up to 1 year if heat-processed	2–3 x 500 ml (17 fl oz/2 cup) jars

We preserve lots of rhubarb in spring, when pear season is finishing and before the stone fruit begins. This recipe is a sweet pickle that is delicious on a cheese plate, with cold meats, or thinly sliced through salads; you could also use this brine for pickling plums, cherries or other red fruits. And once you've eaten all your pickles, remember to save the brine — it becomes an amazing full-flavoured syrup that's great in cocktails, dressings, marinades and not-so-sweet desserts.

PICKLED RHUBARB

Sterilise your jars and lids (see page 212).

Meanwhile, trim the rhubarb stalks, making sure there are no green leaves attached. Cut the stalks into lengths to fit the jars.

Make your brine by combining the vinegar, sugar, water and honey in a non-reactive, medium-sized saucepan. Place over low heat and stir to dissolve the sugar and honey. Add the ginger and slowly bring to simmering point. Turn off the heat and let the flavours infuse the vinegar.

When the jars are cool enough to handle, bring your brine back to simmering point. Using small clean tongs or clean hands, add some of the ginger from the brine to each jar, along with 2 orange peel strips, 4 allspice berries and 4 peppercorns. Carefully pack the rhubarb into the jars, then pour in the hot brine, making sure the rhubarb is completely submerged under the vinegar.

Remove any air bubbles by gently tapping each jar on the work surface and sliding a clean butter knife or chopstick around the inside to release any hidden air pockets. Wipe the rims of the jars with paper towel or a clean damp cloth and seal immediately.

Leave to cool on the benchtop, then store in a cool, dark place for up to 2–3 months (or in the fridge to help maintain a firm texture). The rhubarb will be ready to eat after 2 weeks, but will be better after 1 month. Once opened, refrigerate and use within 2 months.

These pickles are delicious with Christmas ham, and make a great Christmas gift, so if you wanted to make lots of these jars, you can heat-process them (see page 211) for 10 minutes when you make them, which will extend their shelf life to up to 1 year. The rhubarb will lose its shape and texture over time, but the flavour will still be amazing!

6–8 rhubarb stalks
500 ml (17 fl oz/2 cups) red wine vinegar
330 g (11½ oz/1½ cups) raw sugar
250 ml (9 fl oz/1 cup) water
2 tablespoons honey
20 g (¾ oz) knob of fresh ginger, washed but not peeled, cut into slices about 1 cm (½ inch) thick

FOR EACH JAR, YOU WILL NEED:
2 strips of orange peel
4 allspice berries
4 peppercorns

PREPARATION TIME	COOKING TIME	SERVES
20 minutes	about 10 minutes	4

Another excellent example of why we love green tomatoes so much. This salad tastes even better the next day, so make extra!

We prepare a lot of kefir at Cornersmith, but if you're not making it at home or can't buy it at your local store, you can use yoghurt or buttermilk instead.

FRIED GREEN TOMATOES WITH HERBED KEFIR

1.2 kg (2 lb 10 oz) green tomatoes,
    sliced 5 mm (¼ inch) thick
80 ml (2½ fl oz/⅓ cup) olive oil
1 teaspoon finely snipped chives
a few oregano leaves

SPICE MIX
½ teaspoon fenugreek seeds
½ teaspoon celery seeds
⅓ teaspoon dill seeds
1½ teaspoons yellow mustard seeds
1–2 bay leaves

HERBED KEFIR
200 ml (7 fl oz) kefir
1 teaspoon chopped tarragon
1 teaspoon chopped dill
1 teaspoon finely snipped chives
pinch of cayenne pepper, or
    to taste
½ Lebanese (short) cucumber,
    very finely diced

Grind all the spice mix ingredients into a coarse 'powder', using a spice grinder or coffee grinder.

Spread the tomato slices on a large plate or platter, season with salt and pepper and dust with half the spice mix. Turn them over, season with more salt and pepper and dust with the remaining spice mix.

Pour the olive oil into a saucepan large enough to fit all the tomato slices in one layer. (If you don't have a pan large enough, you can cook the tomatoes in several batches.) Heat the oil over medium–high heat, then add the tomato slices, in a single layer. Reduce the heat to medium–low and fry for 4–5 minutes, or until golden brown underneath.

Turn the tomato slices over, put the lid on and braise for another 3–4 minutes, or until the tomatoes are cooked but still retain their shape. Turn the heat off and set aside to cool.

For the herbed kefir, pour the kefir into a bowl and stir in the herbs and cayenne pepper. Fold the diced cucumber through. Season with salt to taste.

Arrange the tomato slices on a large serving platter and drizzle the dressing over them. Serve garnished with the chives and oregano.

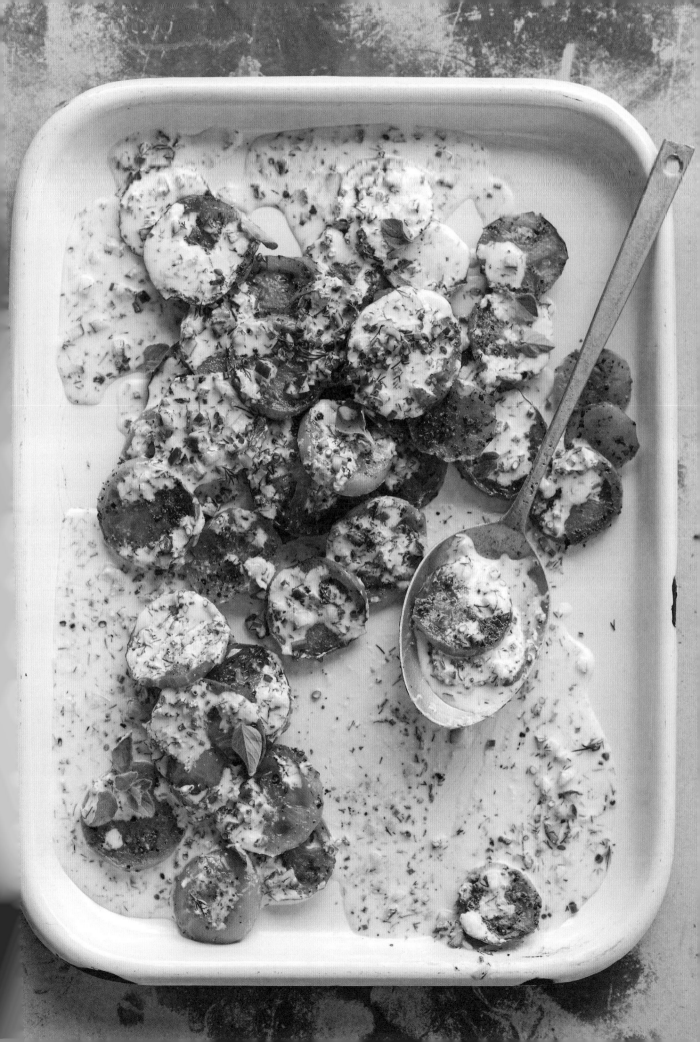

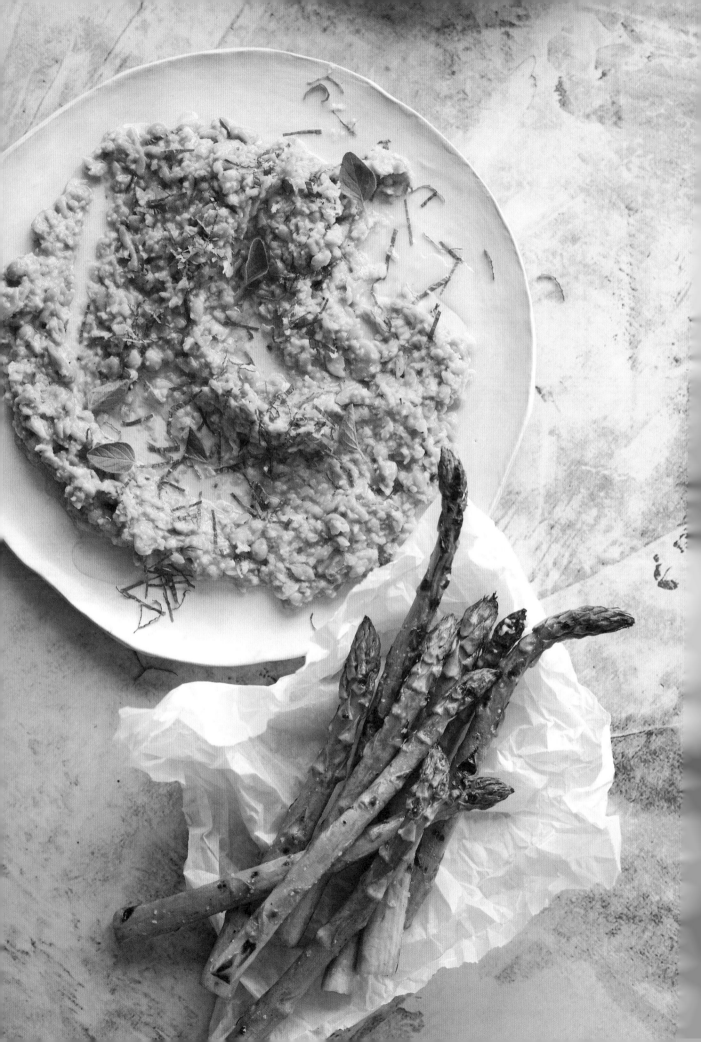

PREPARATION TIME	COOKING TIME	SERVES
20 minutes	15 minutes	4

Not really a salad, but a great way to enjoy all the best spring produce — broad beans, peas, asparagus and mint! — on one plate. To make this mash or dip a bit richer, you can add a small amount of crumbled feta cheese or fresh ricotta; just be careful with your salt seasoning.

MINTY BROAD BEAN & PEA MASH WITH GRILLED ASPARAGUS SOLDIERS

Heat a barbecue or chargrill pan to medium—high.

Meanwhile, trim the woody ends from the asparagus and reserve them for quick pickling (see page 162). Place the asparagus spears in a bowl, add the 2 teaspoons of olive oil, season with salt and pepper and gently mix until coated.

Barbecue or chargrill the asparagus spears for 2—3 minutes, turning them around from time to time so they colour evenly. You want them still a bit crunchy in the middle, for scooping up the mash later on. Set aside.

Bring a medium—large saucepan of salted water to the boil. Blanch the peas for 30—60 seconds, then remove with a slotted spoon. Refresh under cold water, then drain.

Bring the water back up to the boil and blanch the broad beans for 1—2 minutes, then refresh under cold water and drain. When the broad beans are cool enough to handle, peel off and discard the outer skin.

Using a large mortar and pestle, pound the garlic cloves with a couple of pinches of salt, into a fine paste. Add the broad beans and roughly mash them — if your mortar is small, you may have to do this in several batches, or you could pulse them in a food processor. Add the peas and roughly mash. (We prefer our mash not too fine and mushy, but yours can be as smooth or chunky as you like.)

Add the 120—150 ml (4—5 fl oz) of olive oil in a very thin stream, then fold through the lemon zest, chilli powder and lemon juice to taste. Adjust the seasoning to taste, then fold the mint and oregano through.

Place the mash in a serving bowl and finish with a little drizzle of extra olive oil. Serve the grilled asparagus on a plate alongside.

The mash is also delicious as a dip, but loses its vibrant colour the longer it stands.

12 asparagus spears
2 teaspoons olive oil
300 g (10½ oz/2 cups) podded fresh peas
400 g (14 oz) podded fresh broad beans
2 garlic cloves, peeled
120—150 ml (4—5 fl oz) olive oil, plus extra for drizzling over the mash
zest and juice of ½—1 lemon, to taste
pinch of chilli powder
1 handful of mint leaves, thinly sliced
1 tablespoon finely chopped oregano

PREPARATION TIME	COOKING TIME	SERVES
30 minutes, plus overnight soaking	1¾ hours, plus 15 minutes resting	4

These tortillas are basically just edible 'plates' for tender tasty black beans and a fresh spring slaw, dressed with chimichurri.

A versatile green sauce of South American origin, chimichurri is normally made with parsley and coriander leaves; at the cafe, we also add our leftover herb stems, as we're always looking for ways to reduce kitchen waste. Chimichurri is an excellent condiment for grilled meats or fish, vegetables, and avocado.

TORTILLAS WITH BLACK BEANS, SPRING SLAW & CHIMICHURRI DRESSING

200 g (7 oz) white cabbage, finely shaved using a mandoline

150 g (5½ oz) snow peas (mangetout), thinly sliced

2 spring onions (scallions), thinly sliced lengthways into long strips

½–¾ cup sliced Quick Pickled Red Onions (page 41), brine drained and reserved; alternatively, use thinly sliced raw red onions

1 large handful of coriander (cilantro) leaves

8 small tortillas, or 4 large ones (we've used large ones in the photo overleaf)

1 avocado, cut into quarters or eighths

4–8 pieces of Turmeric Pickled Mango (page 42), to garnish (optional)

Cornersmith Chimichurri (see opposite page), to serve

FOR THE BEANS

125 g (4½ oz/⅔ cup) dried black beans, soaked in plenty of cold water overnight

2–3 allspice berries

2 pinches of cumin seeds

2 pinches of coriander seeds

½ white onion, chopped

1 garlic clove, crushed

1 bay leaf

¼ teaspoon salt

2 teaspoons red wine vinegar

CHIMICHURRI DRESSING

2 tablespoons Cornersmith Chimichurri (see opposite page)

2 tablespoons brine from the Quick Pickled Red Onions on page 41; alternatively, use red wine vinegar mixed with a pinch of sugar

2 teaspoons dijon mustard

2 teaspoons warm water

80 ml (2½ fl oz/⅓ cup) olive oil

Start by preparing the beans; for convenience, they can be cooked a day ahead if needed.

Rinse and drain the beans, place them in a saucepan and cover with double their height of water. Add the spices, onion, garlic and bay leaf and bring slowly to the boil. Reduce the heat to low, then simmer for 1–1½ hours, or until cooked but not mushy.

Turn off the heat, stir in the salt and vinegar, then allow the beans to sit for about 15 minutes. Drain the beans and set aside.

Meanwhile, prepare the dressing. In a small jar, combine the chimichurri, pickling brine, mustard and water. Season with salt and pepper, add the olive oil, put the lid on and shake well to combine. Set aside.

In a large bowl, combine the cabbage, snow peas, spring onion, pickled onions and half the coriander. Add the black beans and dressing and mix together very gently.

Divide the salad mixture into four equal portions. Arrange each portion on one large or two small tortillas. Garnish each portion with avocado, pickled mango and a dollop of chimichurri sauce. Garnish with the remaining coriander and serve.

CORNERSMITH CHIMICHURRI

Save your leftover herb stems, keeping them in an airtight container in the fridge until you collect enough for this and other recipes.

Gather together about 80–85 g (3 oz) mixed coriander (cilantro), parsley and dill stems and/or leaves. Wash well, drain and dry.

Place in a food processor with ½ teaspoon lightly toasted cumin seeds, 1 crushed garlic clove, 1½ tablespoons red wine vinegar, ¼ teaspoon salt and a pinch of chilli flakes.

With the motor running, slowly add 100 ml (3½ fl oz) olive oil until combined. Adjust the seasoning to taste.

The chimichurri will keep in the fridge, with a layer of olive oil on top, for up to 1 week.

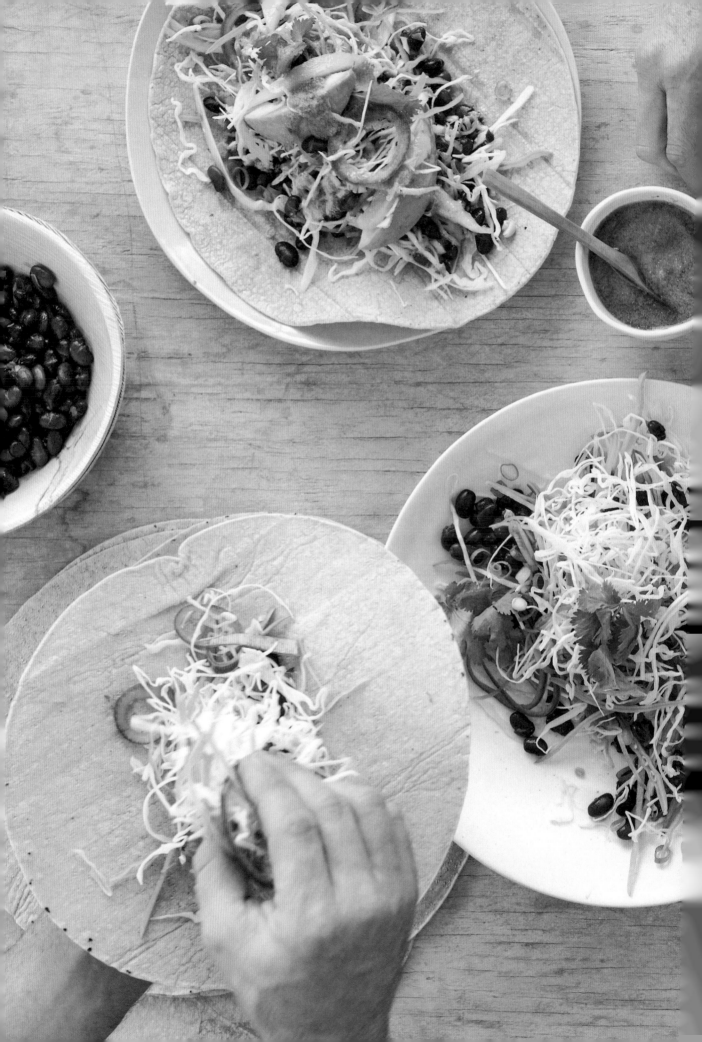

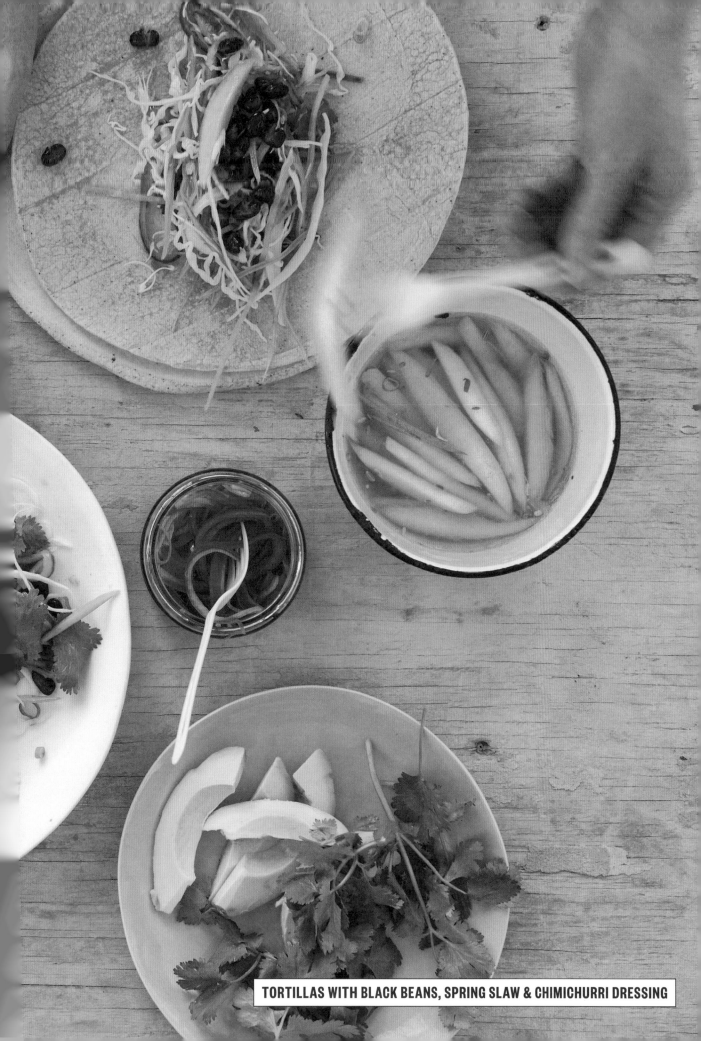

TORTILLAS WITH BLACK BEANS, SPRING SLAW & CHIMICHURRI DRESSING

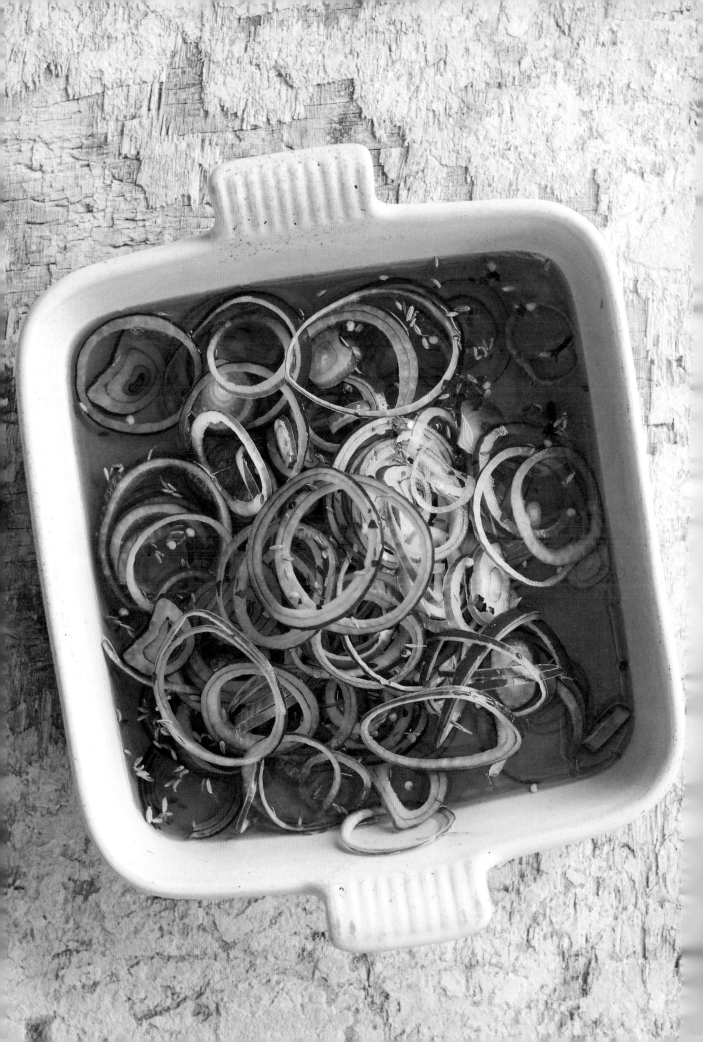

PREPARATION TIME	STORAGE	MAKES
15 minutes, plus 30 minutes salting	up to 1 month	1 x 500 ml (17 fl oz/2 cup) jar or container

These quick and easy pickled onions are great tossed through salads, and on tortillas and burgers. Make them for your next barbecue and everyone will be very impressed that you pickle. They'll last for several weeks in the fridge.

QUICK PICKLED RED ONIONS

Make your brine by combining the vinegar, sugar, salt and water in a non-reactive, medium-sized saucepan. Place over low heat and stir to dissolve the sugar and salt. Add the spices and chilli flakes and slowly bring to simmering point. Turn the heat off and let the brine cool and the flavours develop a little.

Meanwhile, thinly slice the onions and place in a clean jar or non-reactive container. Sprinkle with a little extra salt and leave to sit for 30 minutes or so, to draw out the excess moisture.

Drain off and discard the excess liquid from the onion slices. Pour the room-temperature brine over the onion, making sure all the slices are submerged.

Cover and store in the fridge for up to 1 month.

375 ml (13 fl oz/1½ cups) red wine vinegar
110 g (3¾ oz/½ cup) raw sugar
1 teaspoon salt, plus extra for sprinkling over the onions
125 ml (4 fl oz/½ cup) water
2 cloves
½ teaspoon fennel seeds
½ teaspoon cumin seeds
½ teaspoon chilli flakes
300 g (10½ oz) red onions

PREPARATION TIME	STORAGE	MAKES
25 minutes, plus 20 minutes sterilising, plus 1 hour salting	up to 3 months	3 x 500 ml (17 fl oz/2 cup) jars

So addictive are these pickles, you'll be lucky if they make it past the first meal. They are delicious with curries, or mixed through Asian-style salads such as the Green Mango & Papaya Salad on page 15, and with the tortillas on page 36.

For a quick and tasty salsa to serve with seafood or tacos, finely dice some of the pickled mango and mix in a small amount of the brine, lots of fresh chopped coriander (cilantro), and fresh chilli to taste.

TURMERIC PICKLED MANGO

2 kg (4 lb 8 oz) unripe mangoes, or green mangoes
1½ tablespoons salt
1 teaspoon fenugreek seeds
1 teaspoon fennel seeds
1 teaspoon cumin seeds
½ teaspoon ground turmeric
1 teaspoon yellow mustard powder
1 teaspoon chilli flakes
400 ml (14 fl oz) white wine vinegar
110 g (3¾ oz/½ cup) sugar
400 ml (14 fl oz) water
6 curry leaves

Peel the mangoes, then cut the flesh into long strips about 1 cm (½ inch) thick. Place in a bowl and sprinkle with the salt. Mix with your hands to evenly coat, then leave to sit for at least an hour, to draw the excess moisture out.

While your mango is salting, sterilise your jars and lids (see page 212).

Meanwhile, in a dry frying pan, lightly toast all the spices over medium heat for 1–2 minutes, or until fragrant, taking care not to burn the fenugreek seeds or they will become bitter.

Make your brine by combining the vinegar, sugar and water in a non-reactive, medium-sized saucepan. Place over low heat and stir to dissolve the sugar, then bring to simmering point. Turn off the heat and allow to cool a little.

When the jars are cool enough to handle, drain off and discard the excess liquid from your mango strips; you can wrap them in paper towel to dry them off a bit.

Put 2 curry leaves and 2 teaspoons of your spice mix into the bottom of each jar. Carefully pack the mango strips in. They will have become quite soft from the salting; you want to get as much as you can into each jar, without squashing or breaking up the mango strips.

Cover with the brine, making sure the mango strips are completely submerged under the vinegar.

Remove any air bubbles by gently tapping each jar on the work surface and sliding a clean butter knife or chopstick around the inside to release any hidden air pockets. Wipe the rims of the jars with paper towel or a clean damp cloth and seal immediately.

We prefer to keep these pickles in the fridge, as the texture seems to deteriorate quite quickly. They're best eaten within 3 months.

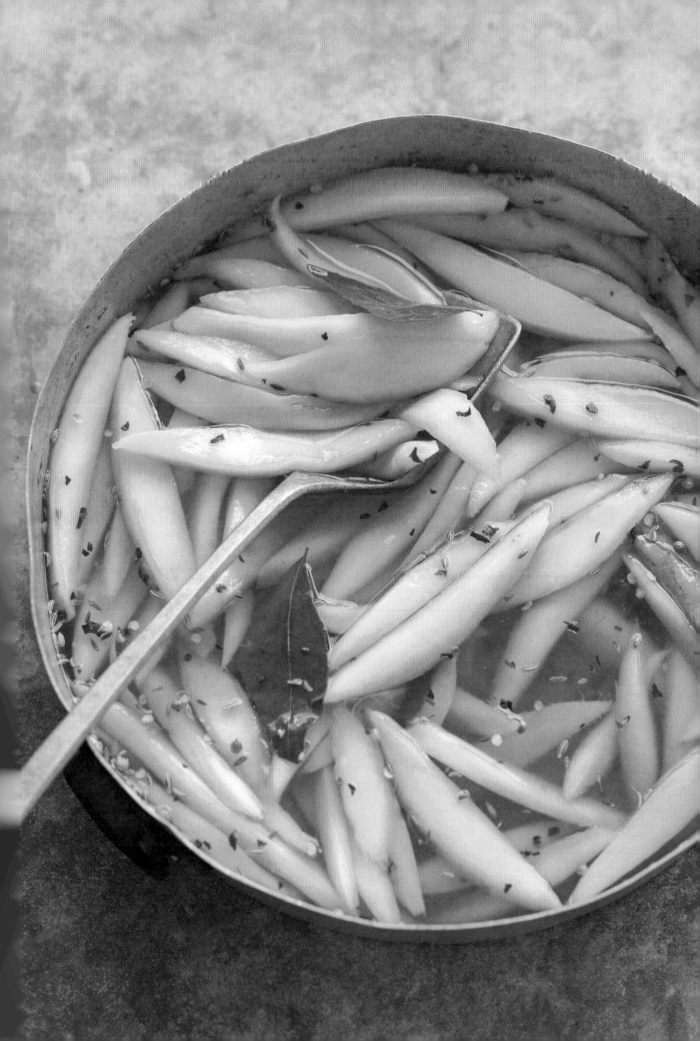

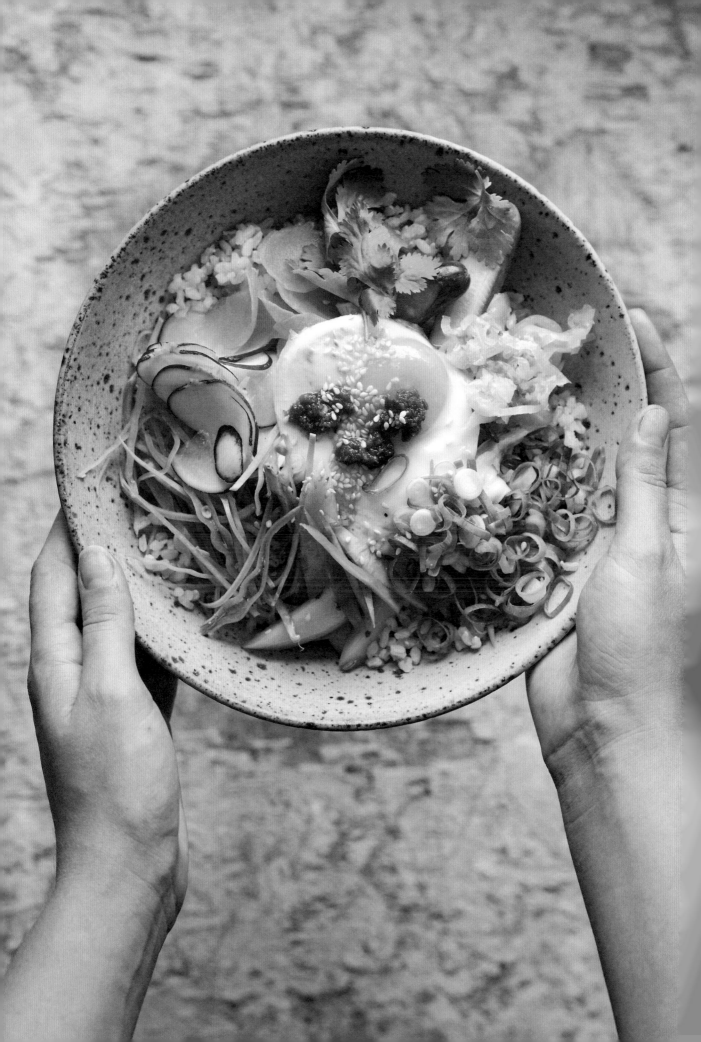

PREPARATION TIME	COOKING TIME	SERVES
15 minutes, plus 20–30 minutes quick pickling	about 1 hour, plus 15 minutes resting	4

This pretty dish often features on our spring menu at our cafes. We borrowed the idea from the Korean bibimbap and turned it into more of a rice salad. It's a great way to combine seasonal raw vegetables and pickles or fermented vegetables from your fridge or pantry into an impressive, quick meal. We've used radishes and snow peas here, but choose whichever raw vegetables you have.

Always serve this with a chilli sauce or sambal — you'll find a few options in the Summer chapter of this book. We don't use imported products at Cornersmith, but other Asian condiments such as fish sauce, soy sauce and Asian chilli pastes would also work well.

CORNERSMITH BIBIMBAP

Wash the rice well, then drain. Place in a saucepan and cover with water, to twice the height of the rice. Add the salt and place over medium–high heat. Bring to the boil, then reduce the heat to low. Cover and very gently simmer for 45 minutes.

Remove the lid and check if the water has been absorbed. If there is more than a tablespoon of water left in the bottom of the pan, drain it off. Take the rice off the heat and let it stand for 10–15 minutes with the lid on.

Place a large frying pan over medium heat. Add the butter. When the butter starts sizzling, crack the eggs into the pan and cook them to your liking; we like the yolks a bit runny, to break them through the rice bowl.

Meanwhile, fluff the rice with a fork and place in four shallow bowls. Arrange your raw, pickled and fermented vegetables in a ring shape around the rice, keeping the middle free for the egg.

When the eggs are done, place one in the centre of each salad. Season with salt. Drizzle the pickling/fermenting brine evenly over the salads. Garnish with the chilli sambal, sesame seeds and coriander and serve.

TIP: If you don't have a pantry full of pickles, use the recipe on page 162 to quick-pickle whatever you have on hand — radishes, carrots, cucumbers, zucchini (courgettes), cauliflower, ginger and green beans would all work well here. Double the recipe of the quick pickling liquid to pickle, for example, 1 small thinly sliced Lebanese (short) cucumber, 4 thinly sliced radishes or 1 small thinly sliced carrot.

250 g (9 oz) medium or short-grain brown rice
1 teaspoon salt
30 g (¾ oz) butter
4 free-range eggs
2 spring onions (scallions), thinly sliced
4 radishes, thinly sliced
10 snow peas (mangetout), cut into very thin strips
pickles, such as ½ cup Zucchini Pickles (page 51) and/or ½ cup Pickled Ginger Carrots (page 153) and/or Turmeric Pickled Mango (page 42)
fermented vegetables, such as ½–¾ cup Kitchen Scrap Sauerkraut (page 192) or Fermented Vegetables (page 46)

TO FINISH
60 ml (2 fl oz/¼ cup) brine from your pickles and ferments
4 teaspoons Chilli Sambal (page 63)
1 teaspoon toasted sesame seeds (see page 206)
½ cup picked coriander (cilantro) leaves (optional)

PREPARATION TIME	FERMENTING TIME	STORAGE	MAKES
20 minutes, plus 20 minutes sterilising	2 days to several weeks	up to 6 months	1–2 x 500 ml (17 fl oz/2 cup) jars

Jaimee Edwards teaches all the fermenting workshops at Cornersmith, and here is her master recipe for brining vegetables. Start with some of the spring vegetables we've suggested here, then experiment with what you have in the fridge or growing in the garden. Fermented vegetables prepared in this way are delicious in salads and on sandwiches — or to eat straight out of the jar.

FERMENTED VEGETABLES

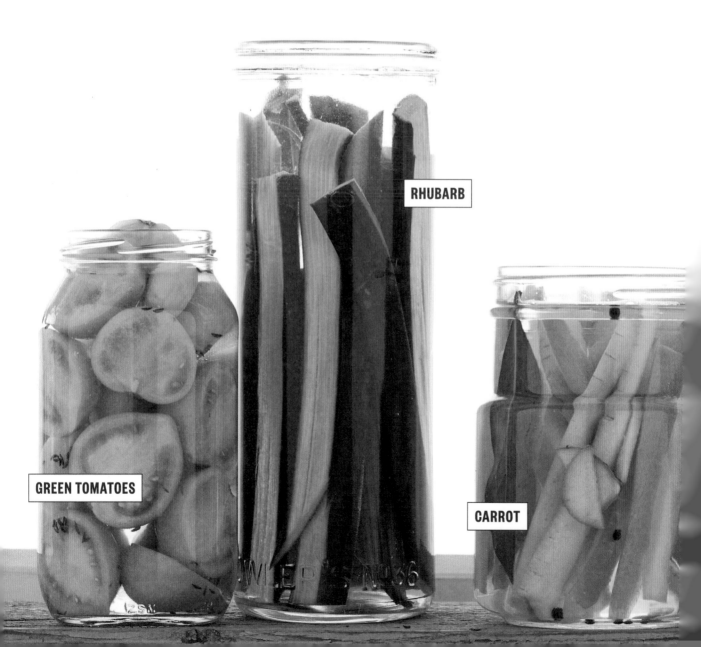

RHUBARB

GREEN TOMATOES

CARROT

Make your salt brine by combining the salt and water in a non-reactive, medium-sized saucepan. Place over low heat and stir to dissolve the salt. Bring to the boil, then turn off the heat and allow to cool to room temperature. (In fermenting never use excessive heat, as this will kill the good bacteria we want to encourage.)

Meanwhile, sterilise your jars and lids (see page 212). Leave to cool to room temperature.

Cut your produce into whatever sizes and shapes you like — remembering that the larger the pieces, the longer they will take to fully ferment.

Pack the vegetables into the jars, to about 1 cm (½ inch) from the top. Pour in your cooled salt brine so that it covers your produce by a few millimetres. Remove any air bubbles by gently tapping the jars on the work surface and sliding a butter knife or chopstick around the inside to release any hidden air pockets. Wipe the rim of the jars with paper towel or a clean damp cloth and seal.

Place your jars out of direct sunlight so the vegetables can begin to ferment. After 2 days, check your ferment to see if the vegetables are at a stage you like. The longer you leave them, the more the flavours will develop. You can leave them to ferment for up to 3 weeks.

Open your jars every few days to 'burp' your ferment — this will release the built-up carbon dioxide, and prevent brine spilling out of the jars. Just be sure to press down your vegetables afterwards, so that the brine is covering the top by at least 1 cm (½ inch).

When your ferments are ready, store them in the refrigerator and eat within 6 months.

1 tablespoon salt
500 ml (17 fl oz/2 cups) water
500 g (1 lb 2 oz) vegetables, such as green (unripe) tomatoes, gherkin cucumbers, carrots, rhubarb stalks, fennel, radishes and/or green chillies

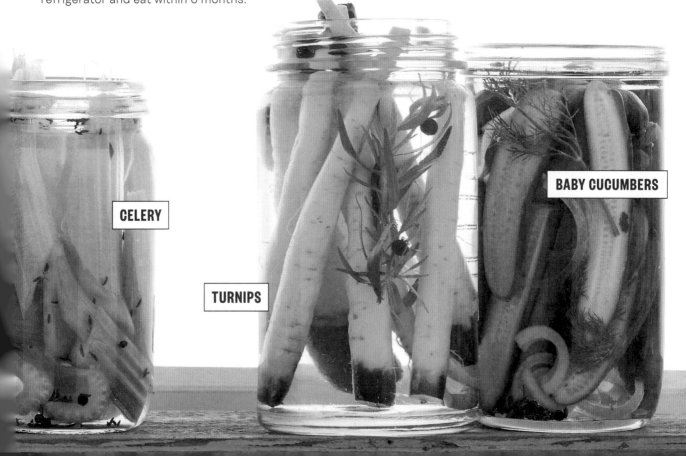

CELERY

TURNIPS

BABY CUCUMBERS

PREPARATION TIME	COOKING TIME	SERVES
20 minutes, plus 20 minutes marinating	about 30 minutes	4

Sabine's brown butter vinaigrette in this potato salad is so good you'll want to bathe in it! Full of flavour, it's an excellent alternative to the more traditional mayonnaise-based dressings, and will be even better if you use a good-quality cultured butter. In fact it's so addictive you may as well make extra and keep it in a jar in your fridge. It will last for up to 5 days, and you can reinvigorate it by placing the jar into a bowl of hot (not boiling!) water and shaking it every now and then until the vinaigrette has emulsified again.

NEW POTATOES WITH PEAS, MINT & BROWN BUTTER VINAIGRETTE

1 kg (2 lb 4 oz) new-season harvest potatoes – a waxy variety, suitable for boiling

300 g (10½ oz) fresh podded peas (frozen are also fine; just pour boiling water over them, leave to thaw for a few minutes, then drain)

60 ml (2 fl oz/¼ cup) hot chicken or vegetable stock

1 large handful of picked mint leaves, torn just before serving

2 tablespoons finely chopped dill

1½ tablespoons finely chopped tarragon

BROWN BUTTER VINAIGRETTE
1 French shallot, finely chopped
1 tablespoon sherry vinegar
60 g (2¼ oz) unsalted butter
2 tablespoons olive oil
2 tablespoons lemon juice
1 tablespoon dijon mustard
pinch of cayenne pepper

Scrub the potatoes and place in a saucepan. Cover with cold water, add a pinch of salt and bring to the boil. Turn the heat down to medium–low and cook for about 20 minutes, or until the potatoes are just cooked. Drain, then set aside to cool down. (New-season potatoes don't need peeling as their skins are very soft and thin.)

Meanwhile, blanch the peas in another saucepan of boiling salted water for 1–2 minutes. Refresh under cold running water, then set aside.

Cut the potatoes into quarters or chunky bite-sized pieces and place in a large bowl. Season with salt and pepper. Pour the hot stock over, cover the bowl with a plate and leave to marinate for 15–20 minutes.

Meanwhile, start preparing the vinaigrette. Combine the shallot and vinegar in a bowl and leave to sit for 5–10 minutes, to mellow the onion flavour.

In a small saucepan, melt the butter over medium heat until it begins to foam. Stir and watch the butter carefully, scraping up any milk solids that stick to the bottom of the pan, until the butter becomes nutty and brown. (Don't let it turn black and bitter!)

Once the butter has the right colour and flavour, add the olive oil and lemon juice directly to the pan. Pour that mixture into a tall container. Add the mustard, and the vinegar and shallot mixture, then blend with a hand-held stick blender until smooth. Add the cayenne pepper and season with salt and pepper.

Gently but thoroughly mix the peas through the marinated potatoes. Add the dressing and gently mix until the vegetables are well coated. Check the seasoning. Add the mint, dill and tarragon and serve immediately, in a large salad bowl.

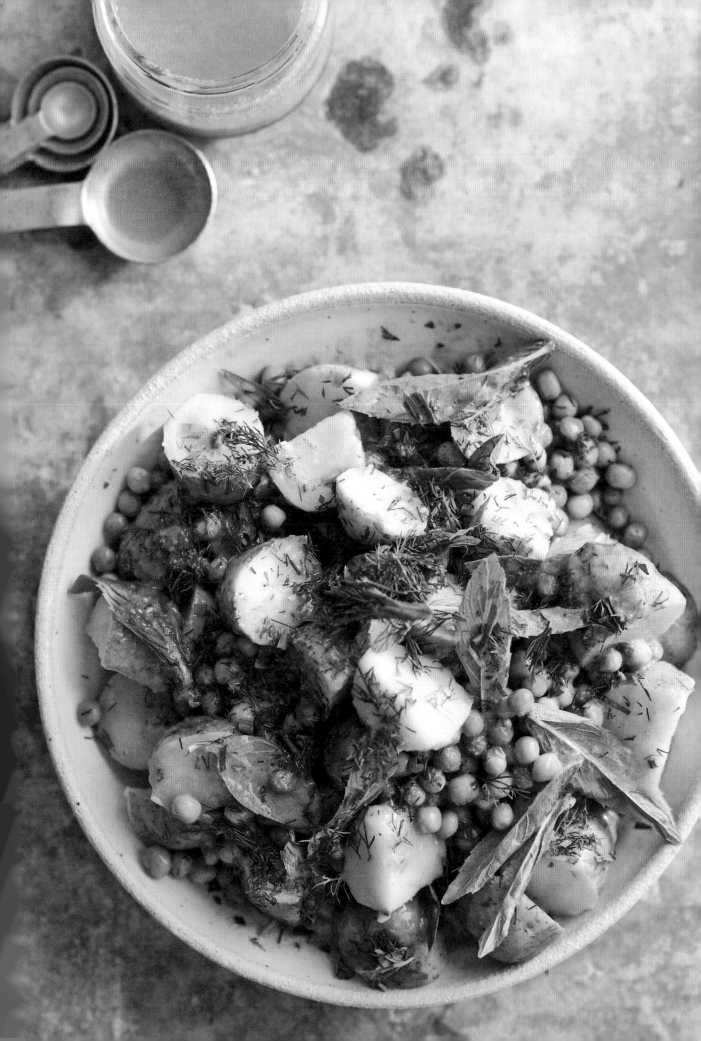

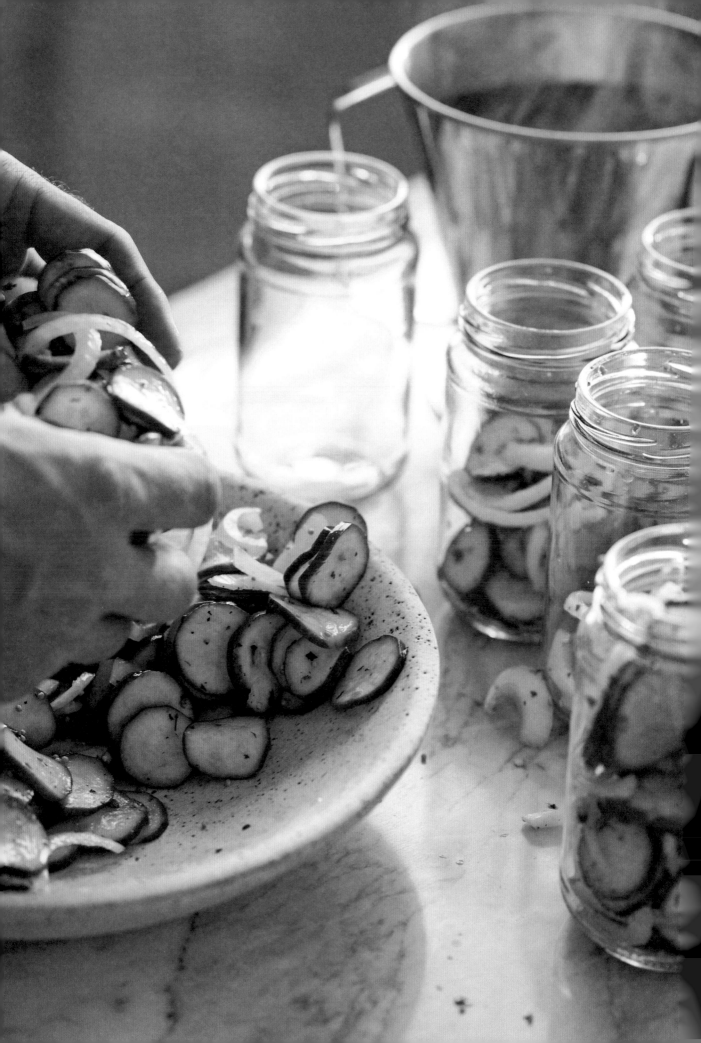

PREPARATION TIME	HEAT-PROCESSING	STORAGE	MAKES
30 minutes, plus 2 hours salting, plus 20 minutes sterilising	10 minutes	up to 2 years	6 x 375 ml (13 fl oz/1½ cup) jars

Make lots of this pickle! It's really delicious and very easy. We made them one year when there weren't many cucumbers around and they've become a staple at Cornersmith. We serve them everywhere you'd use a classic bread and butter pickle. You can leave the chilli out, or add more if you like your pickles hot.

Be sure you don't overpack these jars. If you squish in too much zucchini, the excess moisture in them will be released and make your vinegar brine too watery to preserve properly. And once you've eaten all the pickles, save the brine to use in salad dressings — just whisk in some olive oil and cracked black pepper.

ZUCCHINI PICKLE WITH CHILLI & MINT

Thinly slice the zucchini, to about the thickness of a coin, and place in a large bowl. Thinly slice the onions and mix thoroughly through the zucchini. Sprinkle with the salt and leave to sit for at least 2 hours, to draw out any excess liquid; the larger the zucchini, the longer the mixture will need to sit.

Transfer the zucchini and onion slices to a colander and leave to sit until the liquid has drained out.

Sterilise your jars and lids (see page 212).

Make your brine by combining the vinegar, water and sugar in a non-reactive, medium-sized saucepan. Place over low heat and stir to dissolve the sugar. Increase the heat and bring to the boil.

Place the onion and zucchini slices in a large bowl. Add the mint and spices, mixing with your hand to evenly disperse them.

When the jars are cool enough to handle, use a pair of small clean tongs or clean hands to carefully pack the zucchini mixture into them, so that each jar is full but not overpacked. Remember the brine needs to cover every slice of zucchini, and if they are packed too tightly the brine cannot coat them evenly. Slowly fill the jars with hot brine until the vegetables are completely covered.

Remove any air bubbles by gently tapping each jar on the work surface and sliding a clean butter knife or chopstick around the inside to release any hidden air pockets. Wipe the rims of the jars with paper towel or a clean damp cloth and seal.

Heat-process (see page 211) for 10 minutes, then store in a cool, dark place for up to 2 years. Once opened, refrigerate and use within 6 months.

2 kg (4 lb 8 oz) small firm zucchini (courgettes)
2 small brown onions
2 teaspoons salt
1 litre (35 fl oz/4 cups) white wine vinegar
500 ml (17 fl oz/2 cups) water
165 g (5¾ oz/¾ cup) sugar
3 teaspoons dried mint
3 teaspoons mustard seeds
2 teaspoons chilli flakes (optional)
2–3 peppercorns per jar

PREPARATION TIME	COOKING TIME	STORAGE	MAKES
30 minutes, plus 20 minutes sterilising, plus 10 minutes heat-processing (optional)	about 1 hour	6 months, or up to 2 years if heat-processed	4 x 300 ml (10½ fl oz) jars

Lovely with cheddar, eggs, or at a barbecue or Christmas lunch, this relish is one of our favourites, and is an excellent one to have stocked in the pantry or to give as gifts.

Roasting the rhubarb really intensifies the flavour, so don't skip this step. It also cuts down on the cooking time, once it's in the pot.

RHUBARB & RED ONION RELISH

1 kg (2 lb 4 oz) rhubarb stalks, washed, trimmed and cut into 5 cm (2 inch) lengths

2 tablespoons caster (superfine) sugar

500 ml (17 fl oz/2 cups) red wine vinegar

80 ml (2½ fl oz/⅓ cup) vegetable oil

500 g (1 lb 2 oz) red onions, thinly sliced

50 g (1¾ oz) knob of fresh ginger, peeled and grated

1 teaspoon ground cumin

1 teaspoon ground coriander

½ teaspoon ground fenugreek

2–3 garlic cloves, crushed

500 g (1 lb 2 oz) apples, peeled and grated

200 g (7 oz/1 cup) brown sugar

½ teaspoon salt

Preheat the oven to 180°C (350°F). Spread the rhubarb evenly over two baking trays. Sprinkle with the caster sugar and 80 ml (2½ fl oz/⅓ cup) of the vinegar. Mix with your hands to combine. Roast the rhubarb for about 20 minutes, or until soft and slightly caramelised.

Meanwhile, heat the vegetable oil in a non-reactive, medium-sized saucepan. Add the onion and sauté over medium heat for about 8 minutes, until soft, translucent and sweet. Add the ginger, spices and garlic and sauté for about 2 minutes, until fragrant, stirring constantly.

Add the roasted rhubarb to the pan, along with the remaining vinegar, grated apple, brown sugar and salt, stirring to combine well. Reduce the heat to low.

Simmer, uncovered, for about 30 minutes, stirring now and then, until the relish is thick and glossy, with no puddles on the surface.

Meanwhile, sterilise your jars and lids (see page 212).

Carefully fill the hot jars with the hot relish. Remove any air bubbles by gently tapping each jar on the work surface and sliding a clean butter knife or chopstick around the inside to release any hidden air pockets. Wipe the rims of the jars with paper towel or a clean damp cloth and seal immediately.

Leave to cool on the benchtop, then store in a cool, dark place for up to 6 months. To extend the shelf life to 2 years, heat-process the jars (see page 211) for 10 minutes.

Once opened, refrigerate and use within 3 months.

TIP: If you have some relish left over after you've filled your jars, store it in an airtight container in the fridge and use within 3 weeks.

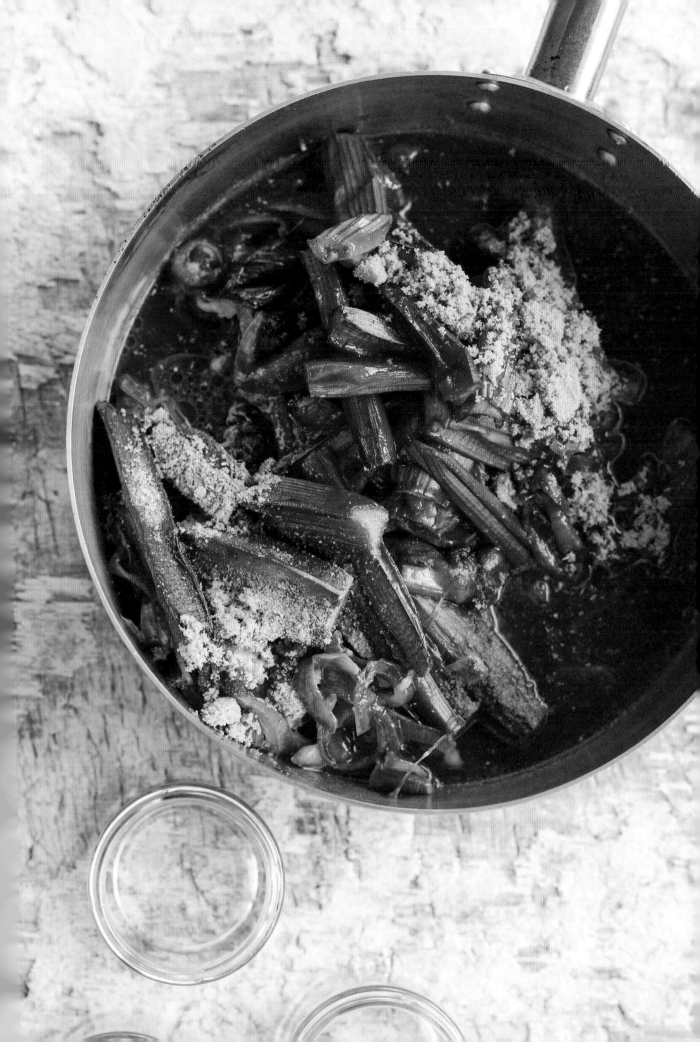

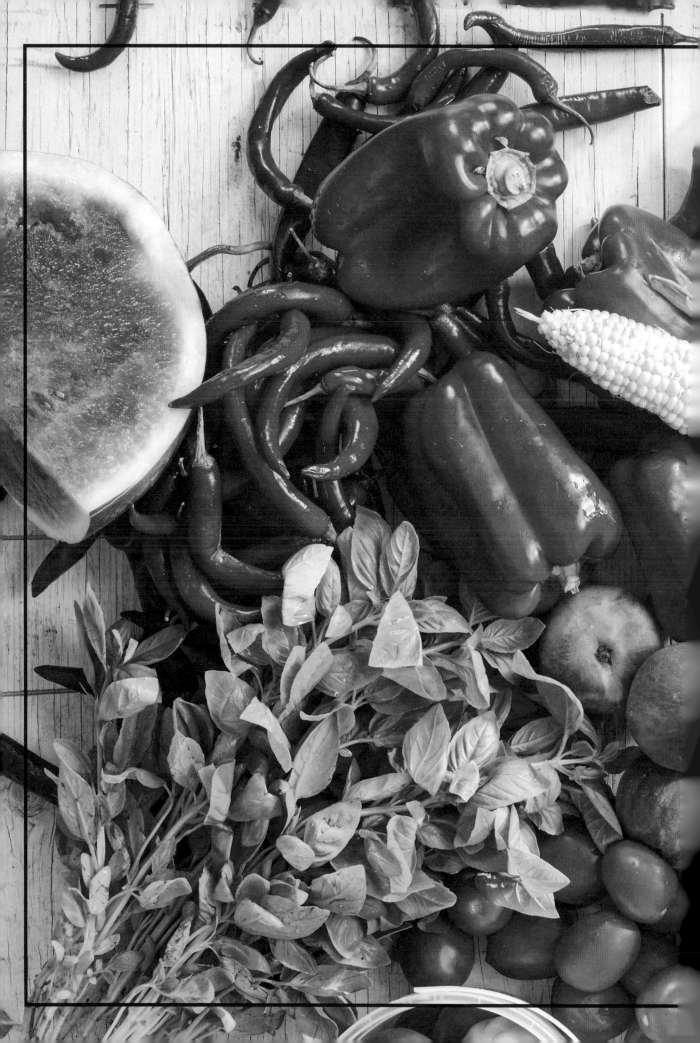

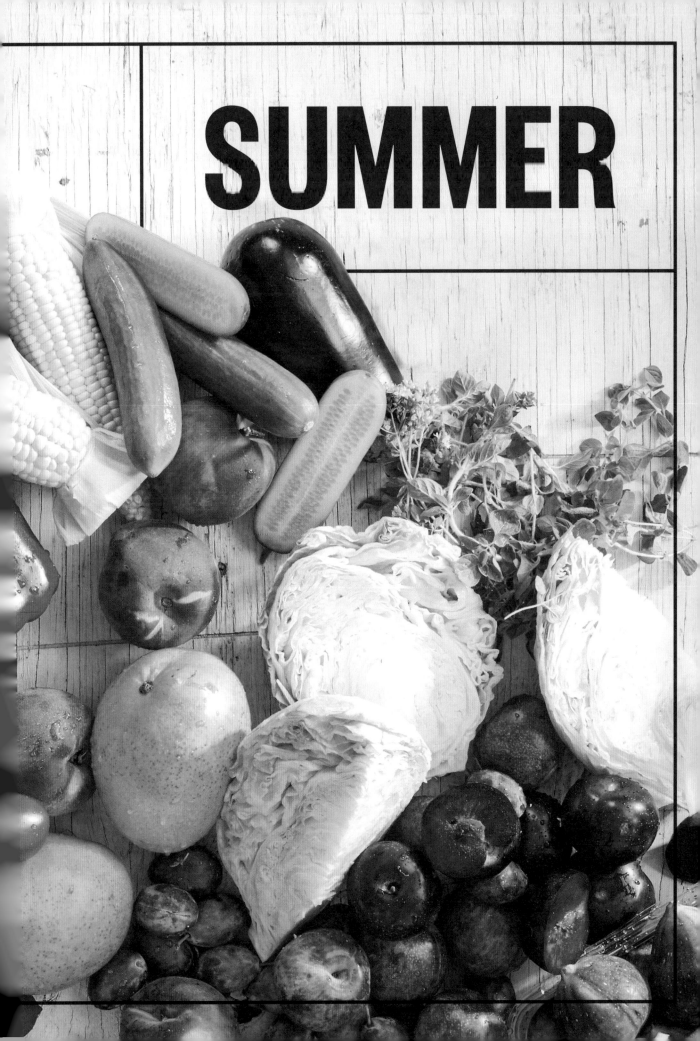

SUMMER

PREPARATION TIME	COOKING TIME	SERVES
25 minutes	40 minutes	4

This is more of a fresh relish than a salad. Rich and flavoursome, it is wonderful with grilled fish and meats, or smeared over ciabatta toasts. The sweetness of the slowly smoked eggplants is balanced by the fruitiness of ripe tomatoes.

Smoking the eggplants is easy and doesn't require a lot of attention. You could also smoke some extra eggplant, cover it with olive oil and keep it in the fridge for up to 5 days, to enjoy with other meals. Or use it in a simple smoky eggplant dip — just scoop out the flesh, drain in a colander for about 10 minutes, then add some crushed garlic, ground cumin, lemon juice, olive oil, salt, pepper and herbs of your liking, and perhaps a splash of tahini and/or yoghurt.

SPICED TOMATO, SMOKY EGGPLANT & PARSLEY

2 medium-sized eggplants
    (aubergines), or 1 large one,
    about 650–700 g (1 lb 7 oz–
    1 lb 9 oz) in total
500 g (1 lb 2 oz) ripe tomatoes
1½ tablespoons olive oil
1½ tablespoons vegetable oil
1½ teaspoons ground cumin
1 large handful of picked flat-leaf
    (Italian) parsley leaves,
    plus extra to serve
juice of 1–2 lemons

Heat a barbecue to medium–high. Prick the eggplant all over with a fork, then place directly on the barbecue. If you have a barbecue with a lid, close the lid, so the eggplant will absorb all the delicious smoky flavours. Cook for about 25–35 minutes, turning every 8–10 minutes, so the skin burns and blisters all over, and the inner flesh collapses fully. When the eggplant is totally charred, allow to cool for about 10 minutes.

Meanwhile, prepare the tomatoes. Cut half into bite-sized pieces, place in a large bowl, season with salt and pepper and set aside. Finely dice the rest.

Heat the olive oil and vegetable oil in a frying pan until quite hot; small bubbles should form around a wooden spoon when you dip it in the oil. (The oil will spit a little when you add the juicy tomatoes, so if you want to avoid a mess in your kitchen, you could place the oiled pan on your barbecue and do this step outside.) Add the diced tomato to the pan, along with the cumin, 1 cup parsley and a pinch of salt. Give a quick stir, being careful to avoid hot splatters. Cook over high heat for 2–3 minutes, until the tomato softens. Remove from the heat and add to the fresh tomatoes in the bowl.

Using a serrated knife, cut the charred eggplant in half lengthways. Scoop out the flesh, avoiding any burnt bits of skin, as they will make the salad taste bitter.

Tear the scooped-out eggplant flesh into bite-sized pieces, and add them to the tomato mixture. Add the lemon juice to taste and adjust the seasoning. Fold some extra parsley through. Serve immediately, on a big plate or in a shallow bowl.

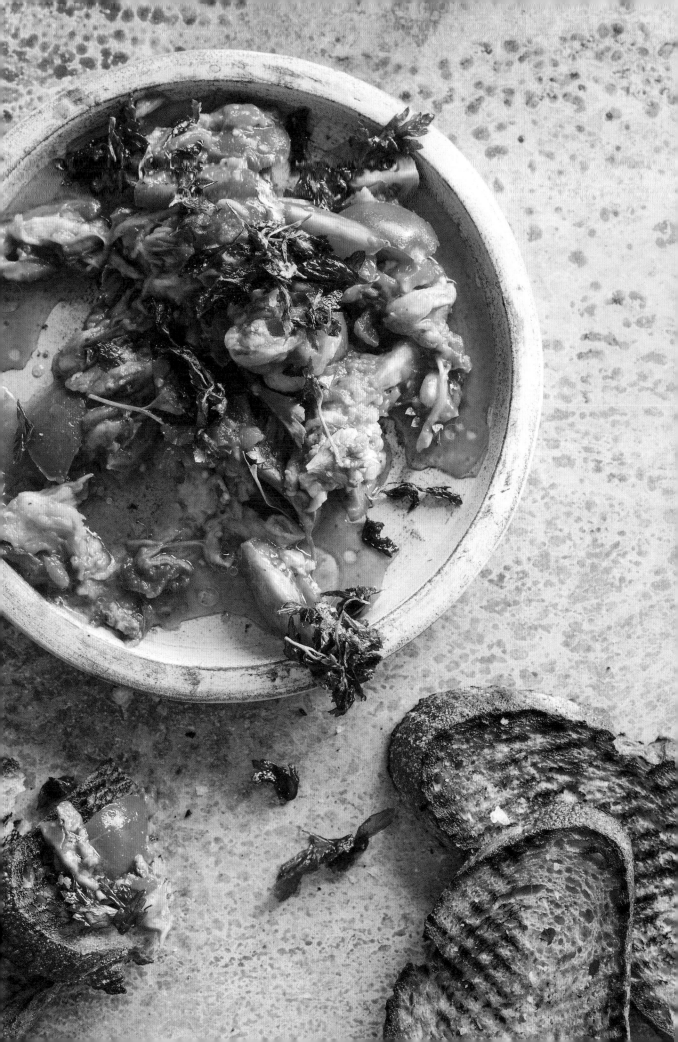

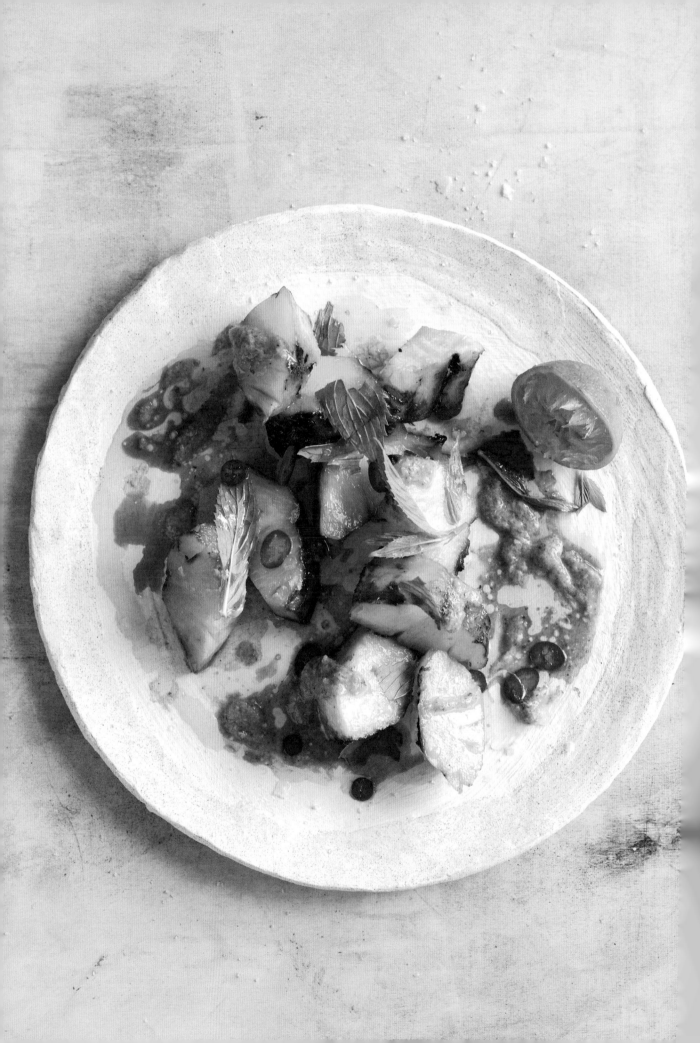

PREPARATION TIME	COOKING TIME	SERVES
15 minutes	20 minutes	4

Grilled pineapple is so delicious! Its sweet acidity balances out the salt and chilli in this summery savoury fruit salad. It is refreshing on its own, but also pairs well with grilled meat or fatty fish. Another great use for the Chimichurri recipe on page 37.

GRILLED PINEAPPLE, SEA SALT, CHILLI, MINT & CHIMICHURRI

Heat a barbecue to medium–low. Grill the pineapple quarters on the barbecue for about 10–15 minutes, turning now and then, until evenly coloured on all sides.

Cut the charred pineapple pieces into bite-sized pieces and place on a serving plate.

Sprinkle with the sea salt, drizzle with the chimichurri dressing, olive oil and citrus juice, then finish with a scattering of chilli and mint.

TIP: Use the pineapple skins to make a pineapple syrup. Make a base sugar syrup, from the Summer Fruit with Mint Stem Syrup recipe on page 77; you might have to multiply the ingredients a few times, but a triple quantity should be enough. When you put the syrup ingredients on the stove, add the finely chopped skins and cores of the pineapple and some spices such as cloves, allspice berries and peppercorns. Simmer over very low heat for 20–30 minutes, then strain out the skins, cores and spices. Check the consistency, and put the syrup back on the stove to reduce further if needed. It can be used to marinate meats for the barbecue, to finish desserts, to use instead of cordials for drinks (with or without alcohol), or simply to drizzle over ice cream. It will keep in a clean container in the fridge for at least 4 weeks.

1 pineapple, about 1.5 kg
    (3 lb 5 oz), cut into quarters,
    skin and core removed (see tip)
pinch of sea salt
2 teaspoons Chimichurri dressing
    (see page 37)
olive oil, for drizzling
juice of 1–2 limes or lemons
½ small red chilli, cut into very
    thin slices
6–8 mint leaves, torn into pieces
    just before serving

PREPARATION TIME	COOKING TIME	STORAGE	MAKES
20 minutes, plus 20 minutes sterilising, plus 10 minutes heat-processing (optional)	about 1¼ hours	3 months, or up to 2 years if heat-processed	4 x 300 ml (10½ fl oz) jars

When mangoes are cheap or you have a neighbourhood mango tree that is dropping fruit faster than you can eat it, make this chutney! It's delicious with curries and seafood and makes a great gift. This one has a bit of heat to it, but you can leave the chilli flakes out if you're after something milder.

MANGO CHUTNEY

1.8–2 kg (4 lb–4 lb 8 oz) sweet, ripe mangoes; you'll need about 1.2 kg (2 lb 10 oz) sliced mango
1 brown onion
1 red onion
80 ml (2½ fl oz/⅓ cup) olive, sunflower or vegetable oil
2 teaspoons salt
1 teaspoon yellow mustard seeds
1 teaspoon brown mustard seeds
1 teaspoon ground coriander
1½ teaspoons ground ginger
1 teaspoon chilli flakes
¼ teaspoon cayenne pepper
300 ml (10½ fl oz) apple cider vinegar
110 g (3¾ oz/½ cup) sugar

Cut the mangoes into 3 cm (1¼ inch) cubes and discard the peel and stones. Very thinly slice the onions.

Measure out the spices and set aside.

Heat the oil in a large non-reactive saucepan. Add the onions and sauté with the salt over medium–low heat for about 8 minutes, until soft and collapsed. Add the spices and stir for a minute or two, until fragrant.

Add the mango and stir until the spices are evenly mixed through. Add the vinegar and sugar, stirring to dissolve the sugar.

Cook over low heat, stirring regularly to make sure the chutney isn't sticking, for up to 1 hour, or until the chutney is glossy and thick, with no puddles of liquid on the surface. Taste and add more spices or salt if needed, then turn off the heat and leave to cool for a minute or two.

Meanwhile, sterilise your jars and lids (see page 212), putting the jars in the oven about 15 minutes before the chutney has finished cooking.

Fill the hot jars with the hot chutney. Remove any air bubbles by gently tapping each jar on the work surface and sliding a clean butter knife around the inside to release any hidden air pockets. Wipe the rims of the jars with paper towel or a clean damp cloth and seal immediately.

Leave to cool on the benchtop, then store in a cool, dark place for up to 3 months. To extend the shelf life to 2 years, heat-process the jars (see page 211) for 10 minutes.

Try to let the chutney sit for 1 month before you eat it. Once opened, refrigerate and use within 3 months.

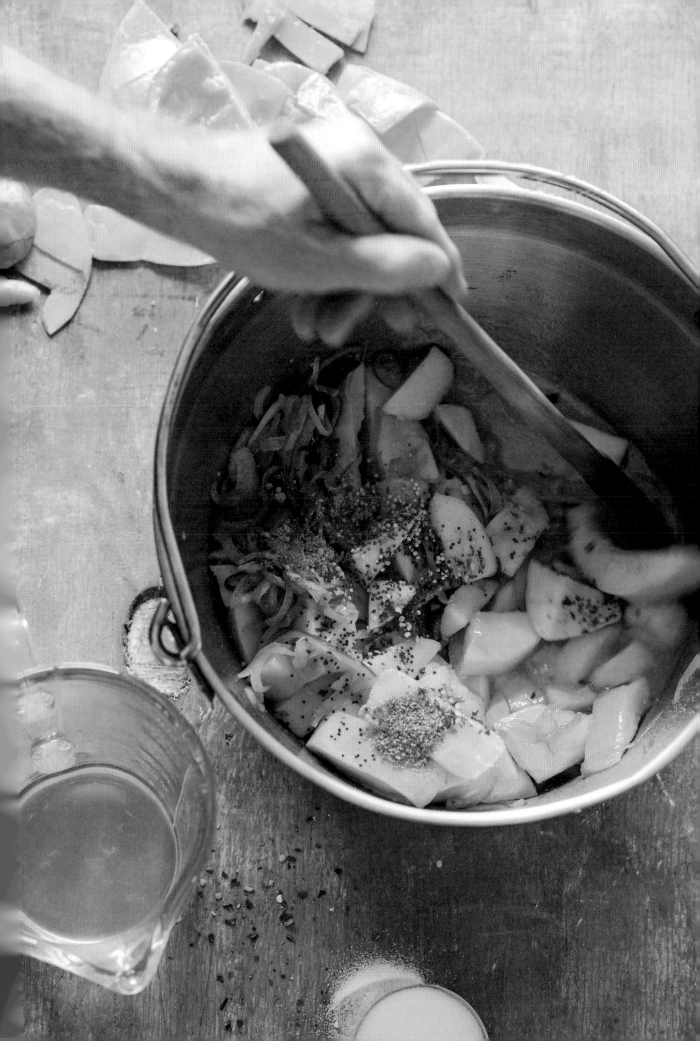

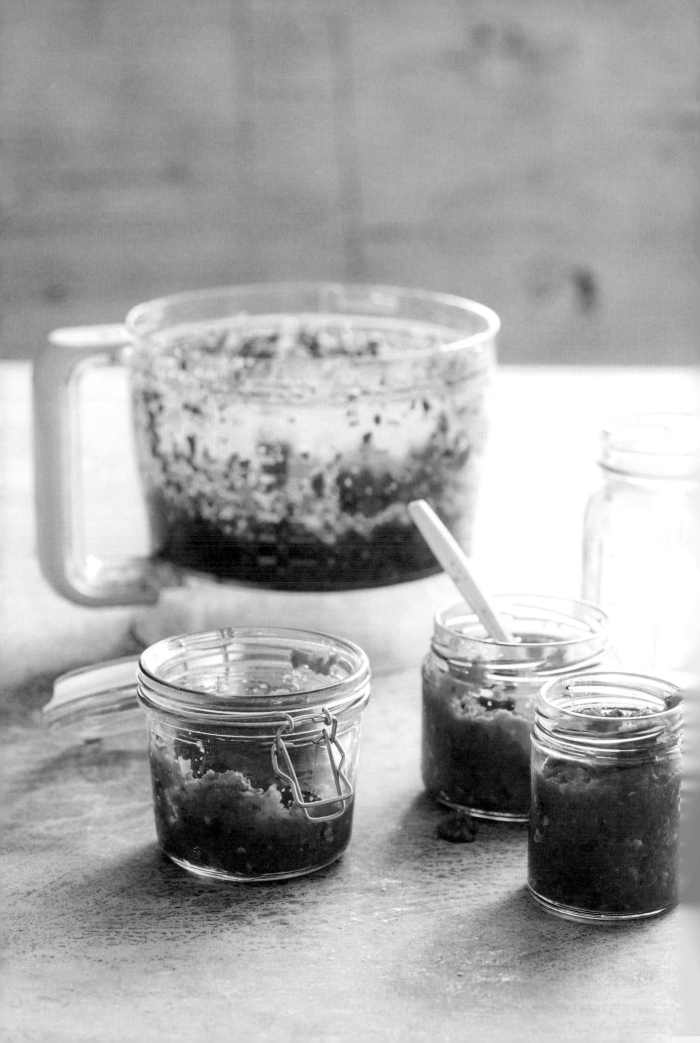

PREPARATION TIME	STORAGE	MAKES
20 minutes, plus 20 minutes sterilising, plus 10 minutes heat-prooooɔing (optional)	3 months, or up to 2 years if heat-processed	4–5 x 375 ml (13 fl oz/1½ cup) jars

We make mountains of this sambal when chilli season is in full swing. It's a staple at Cornersmith, and in all our fridges at home. So quick and easy to make, it gives tacos, rice dishes, marinades and breakfast eggs a good hit of heat.

We use carrot as a base in this recipe as it adds sweetness and gives the sambal a fantastically bright colour, but you could experiment with other bases such as green mango or pineapple. Try green or yellow chillies too.

With fruit-based sambals, you may need to add more vinegar to loosen them. Keep tasting and adjusting the sugar/salt ratio until you're happy with the flavour.

CHILLI SAMBAL

Sterilise your jars and lids (see page 212).

Roughly chop the chillies, carrot, ginger and garlic cloves. Place in a food processor with the sugar and salt and blitz for 5 minutes. Slowly pour in the vinegar until your sambal has a smooth consistency; you may need to adjust the quantity.

When the jars are cool enough to handle, pack the sambal into the jars, pressing down firmly to make sure the chilli paste is covered in a thin layer of liquid.

Remove any air bubbles by gently tapping each jar on the work surface and sliding a clean butter knife or chopstick around the inside to release any hidden air pockets. Wipe the rims of the jars with paper towel or a clean damp cloth and seal immediately.

You can store the sambal in the fridge for up to 3 months, or heat-process the jars (see page 211) for 10 minutes and store in a cool, dark place for up to 2 years.

Once opened, refrigerate and use within 3 months.

TIP: If your chillies are extra hot, you can always change the ratio of the sambal. Try 500 g (1 lb 2 oz) carrot to 500 g (1 lb 2 oz) chillies – or even 750 g (1 lb 10 oz) carrot to 250 g (9 oz) chillies.

750 g (1 lb 10 oz) long mild red chillies
250 g (9 oz) carrot
50 g (1¾ oz) knob of fresh ginger
4 garlic cloves
55 g (2 oz/¼ cup) sugar
1 tablespoon salt
185 ml (6 fl oz/¾ cup) white wine vinegar

PREPARATION TIME	COOKING TIME	SERVES
15 minutes	15 minutes	4

Strictly speaking, this isn't really a salad — but it's still a bit of a summer essential, warmly welcomed at any barbecue.

WHOLE GRILLED CORN, WITH MISO & LIME AIOLI & BASIL

4 corn cobs, in their husks
1 tablespoon olive oil, plus extra
    for drizzling
¼ teaspoon Chilli Sambal
    (page 63)
1 teaspoon miso paste
juice of ½ lime
2 tablespoons Aioli (page 85)
1 small handful of picked basil
    leaves
1 lime, cut into wedges, to serve

Heat a barbecue to medium–high.

Remove the husks from the corn cobs; reserve them for another use (see tip). Remove any silky threads and place the cobs in a bowl. Add the olive oil, season with salt and pepper and toss until the cobs are evenly coated with the oil and seasoning.

Place the cobs on the barbecue and grill them, turning often, for about 8–10 minutes, until golden brown all over. Remove from the heat and set aside to cool.

In a small bowl, combine the chilli sambal and miso paste until smooth, adding a little lime juice to taste. Mix the aioli through, then check the seasoning.

Cut the corn cobs in half, if you like, and place on a large plate. Evenly drizzle the remaining lime juice over the top, then the miso and lime aioli and some extra olive oil. Garnish with the basil and serve with lime wedges.

TIP: Don't throw the corn husks out. Grill them on your barbecue until charred and black, then keep them under vegetable oil to infuse for a few weeks. This will create a really sweet, corn-flavoured oil, which you can use in salad dressings, for cooking meat or vegetables, or when making your next mayonnaise.

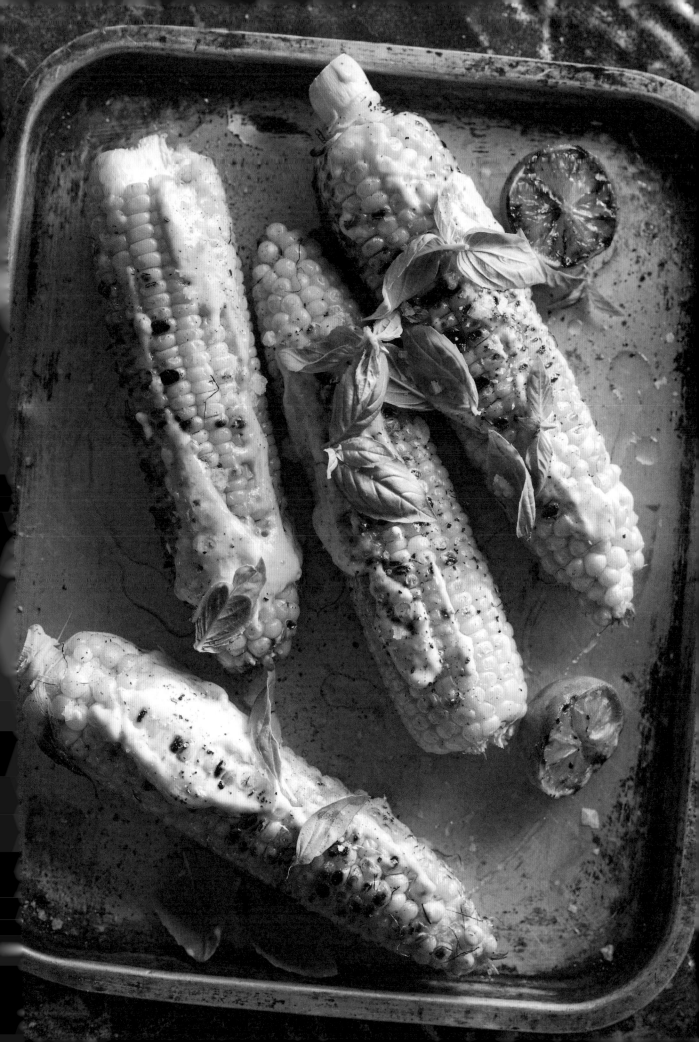

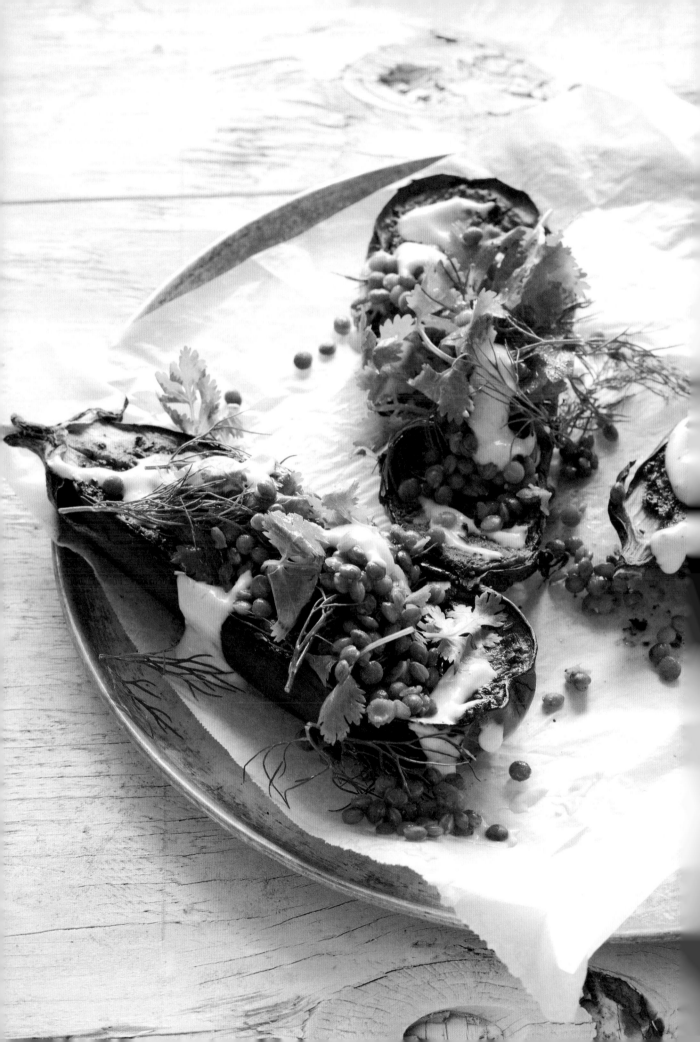

PREPARATION TIME	COOKING TIME	SERVES
25 minutes, plus at least 8 hours soaking and 45 minutes salting	25 minutes	4

An old-time favourite in our cafes, with a distinctly Middle Eastern flavour, this salad makes a lovely vegetarian summer meal. For a dairy-free version, leave the yoghurt out of the dressing and add a splash of warm water and lemon juice.

SPICED EGGPLANT WITH LENTIL & HERB SALAD & TAHINI YOGHURT

Using a sharp knife, cut the eggplants in half lengthways, then score the flesh with deep diagonal lines, about 2 cm (¾ inch) apart, at 90 degrees to each other, so you end up with a diamond pattern, without cutting through the skin.

Sprinkle the cut side of the eggplants with salt and leave to stand for 30–45 minutes.

Meanwhile, rinse the soaked lentils and place in a saucepan with about 500 ml (17 fl oz/2 cups) fresh water. Add the onion halves, garlic, peppercorns, cloves and bay leaf. Slowly bring to a simmer over medium heat, then leave to simmer for 15–20 minutes, or until the lentils are just soft but still retain their shape. Turn off the heat, add the salt, then cover and leave to stand for 10–15 minutes, for the lentils to absorb the salt. Set aside in their cooking liquid until needed.

When the eggplant is nearly ready, preheat the oven to 180°C (350°F). Line a baking dish with baking paper.

In a small bowl, mix together the olive oil, ground spices, garlic and salt. Rinse the eggplants, then give them a firm squeeze to get rid of any excess moisture. Dry well and brush the spiced oil over the cut sides.

Place in the baking dish and bake for 15–20 minutes, or until cooked through and golden brown on top. Set aside to cool a little.

To make the tahini yoghurt, combine the tahini and chimichurri in a small bowl, mixing until smooth. Fold the yoghurt through and check the seasoning.

Drain the lentils and place in a bowl. Add the vinegar, olive oil, and salt and pepper to taste. Tear up the herbs and add half to the lentils. Gently mix until dressed.

Place an eggplant half on each serving plate. Reserve 2 tablespoons of the tahini yoghurt and spread the rest evenly over the eggplant. Arrange the lentil salad on top, then garnish with the remaining herbs and tahini yoghurt. Finish with a sprinkling of sesame seeds, if using, and a drizzle of olive oil.

2 medium-sized eggplants (aubergines), about 440 g (15½ oz) each
2 tablespoons olive oil, plus extra for drizzling over the salad
1 teaspoon garam masala
½ teaspoon ground cumin
¼ teaspoon ground allspice
¼ teaspoon sweet paprika
2 garlic cloves, crushed
1–2 pinches of salt
1 teaspoon black or white sesame seeds (optional)

LENTIL & HERB SALAD
100 g (3½ oz) small brown lentils, soaked in water for 8 hours, or overnight
1 small onion, cut in half
1 garlic clove, peeled
3–4 black peppercorns
3 cloves
1 bay leaf
½ teaspoon salt
1 tablespoon apple cider vinegar
2 tablespoons olive oil
1 small handful coriander (cilantro)
1 small handful picked parsley, dill or chervil leaves

TAHINI YOGHURT
3 teaspoons tahini
2 teaspoons Chimichurri dressing (page 37)
100 g (3½ oz) natural unsweetened yoghurt

PREPARATION TIME	COOKING TIME	STORAGE	MAKES
20 minutes, plus 20 minutes sterilising, plus 15 minutes heat-processing (optional)	30 minutes	3 months, or up to 1 year if heat-processed	3–4 x 500 ml (17 fl oz/2 cup) jars

We roast many different kinds of vegetables before we pickle them, including eggplants, red capsicums, cauliflower, zucchini and fennel. The roasting, pickling and added oil ends up making a more antipasto style of pickle, like those you buy from the delicatessen. They're perfect for picnics!

This is also a good way to use up any excess vegies you have in the fridge at the end of the week. For crunchy pickles, you need fresh, crispy vegetables — but for this style of pickling, eggplants that are going a little soft or zucchini that are a bit wrinkly will work well.

ROASTED PICKLED EGGPLANT

2 kg (4 lb 8 oz) medium-sized
   eggplants (aubergines)
60 ml (2 fl oz/¼ cup) extra virgin
   olive oil or vegetable oil
1 tablespoon salt
750 ml (26 fl oz/3 cups) white
   wine vinegar
375 ml (13 fl oz/1½ cups) water
110 g (3¾ oz/½ cup) sugar

FOR EACH JAR, YOU WILL NEED:
½ teaspoon black peppercorns
½ teaspoon chilli flakes, or
   1 whole red chilli
2 oregano sprigs
2 garlic cloves, peeled
extra virgin olive oil or vegetable
   oil, for covering the eggplant

Preheat the oven to 200°C (400°F). Cut the top and bottom off each eggplant, then cut each eggplant lengthways into quarters. Place on a baking tray, drizzle with the olive oil and sprinkle with the salt. Roast for 20 minutes, or until the eggplant is starting to soften and is browning at the edges.

Sterilise your jars and lids (see page 212).

Make your brine by combining the vinegar, water and sugar in a non-reactive, medium-sized saucepan. Place over low heat and stir to dissolve the sugar. Increase the heat and allow to simmer for 5 minutes.

When the jars are cool enough to handle, add the peppercorns and chilli flakes to each jar.

Strain any excess liquid from the eggplant, then pack each jar half full with eggplant. Add the oregano sprigs and garlic cloves, then pack in the remaining eggplant.

Pour the hot brine over the eggplant, filling each jar only three-quarters of the way up. Remove any air bubbles by gently tapping each jar on the work surface and sliding a clean butter knife or chopstick around the inside of the jars to release any hidden air pockets.

Pour in enough olive oil to completely cover the eggplant. Wipe the rims of the jars with paper towel or a clean damp cloth and seal immediately.

Leave to cool on the benchtop, then store in the fridge for up to 3 months, or heat-process the jars (see page 211) for 15 minutes and store in a cool, dark place for up to 1 year.

Once opened, refrigerate and use within 2 months.

If the oil solidifies in the fridge, leave the jar at room temperature for an hour or so before serving.

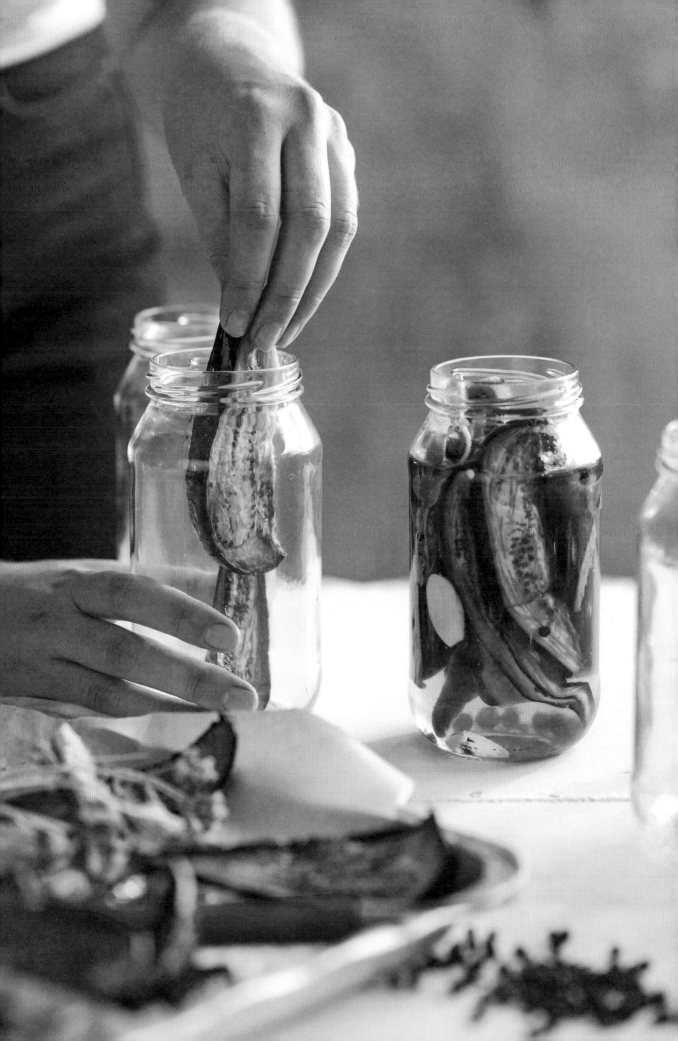

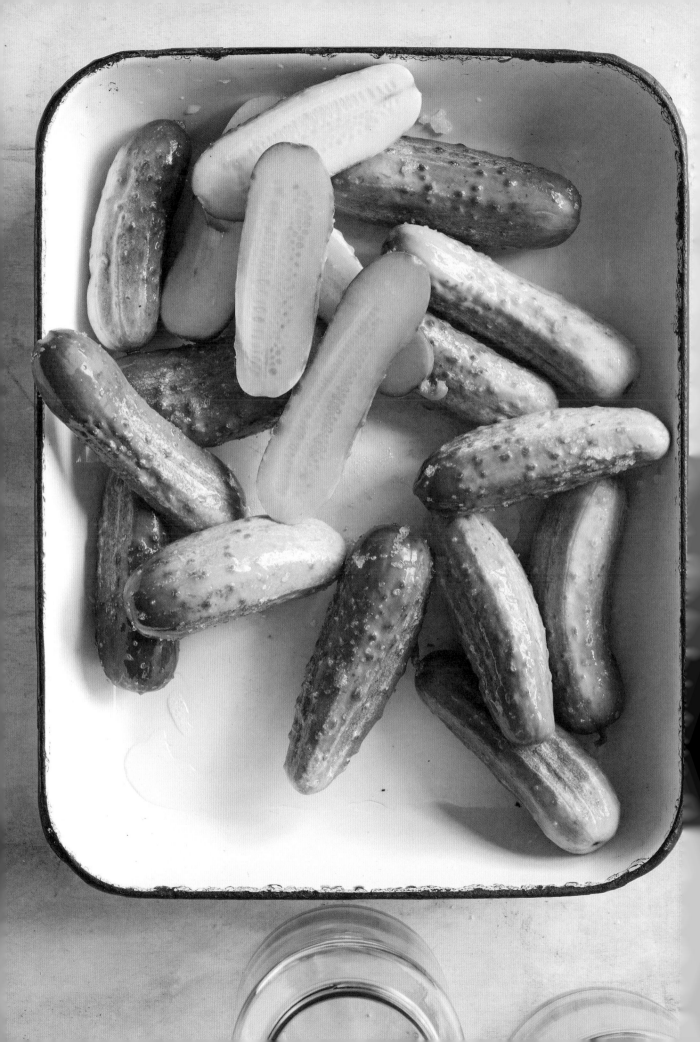

PREPARATION TIME	HEAT-PROCESSING	STORAGE	MAKES
20 minutes, plus overnight salting, plus 20 minutes sterilising	15 minutes	up to 2 years	2 x 750 ml (26 fl oz) jars

This is a classic vinegar-based dill pickle. We often get asked where to find gherkins, as they're not usually available in supermarkets. The only reason you don't see them in supermarkets is that no one buys them raw. If you have a chat with your local greengrocer in early summer, they'll be able to order a box for you.

Make sure you don't skip the overnight salting step of this recipe. It makes your pickles stay crunchy and fresh. You can add other flavourings you like to the jars — bay leaves, thyme, lemon peel, peppercorns, caraway and chilli are all delicious. If you're growing dill or fennel at home, let some go to seed, and use the flowers in your jars instead of the dried dill.

GHERKINS

Wash the gherkins and remove any blemished ends or flowers that are still attached. If your gherkins are different sizes, cut the big ones in half so they're all similar in size.

Put the gherkins in a non-reactive bowl and sprinkle with the salt. Leave to sit overnight in the fridge. You need to do this in order to draw out excess moisture, or your brine will be too watery. It also helps your pickles keep their crunch.

The next day, strain off and discard any liquid.

Sterilise your jars and lids (see page 212).

Make your brine by combining the vinegar, water and sugar in a non-reactive, medium-sized saucepan. Place over low heat and stir to dissolve the sugar. Increase the heat and bring to the boil.

When the jars are cool enough to handle, add the spices to each jar. Carefully pack the gherkins vertically in the jars. Add the hot brine to completely cover the gherkins. Then add a few more gherkins, laying them horizontally on top to hold the other gherkins down under the brine.

Remove any air bubbles by gently tapping each jar on the work surface and sliding a clean butter knife or chopstick around the inside to release any hidden air pockets. You may need to add more brine to ensure the gherkins are completely submerged. Wipe the rims of the jars with paper towel or a clean damp cloth and seal.

Heat-process (see page 211) for 15 minutes, then leave to sit for at least 2 months before opening. They will keep for up to 2 years, stored in a cool, dark place.

Once opened, refrigerate and use within 6 months.

1.2 kg (2 lb 10 oz) small gherkins (pickling cucumbers)
1 tablespoon salt
625 ml (21½ fl oz/2½ cups) white wine vinegar
310 ml (10¾ fl oz/1¼ cups) water
55–110 g (2–3¾ oz/¼–½ cup) caster (superfine) sugar, depending on how sweet you like your pickles

FOR EACH JAR, YOU WILL NEED:
¼ teaspoon whole black peppercorns
1 teaspoon dill seeds
¼ teaspoon dried dill
1 teaspoon mustard seeds

FLAVOURED SALTS

Flavoured salts are a staple in Cornersmith kitchens and on our retail shelves. We make them as a way to use up excess citrus skins, herbs and chillies, but they also happen to be delicious for seasoning vegetables and meats before grilling, for roasting potatoes, in salad dressings, and even for pickling.

Flavoured salts are so easy to make. You just need to make sure whatever aromatic you are mixing into your salt is completely dried or dehydrated. Any moisture left in your herbs or chillies will cause the salt to clump together, and potentially allow mould to develop.

Also, try to use pure granulated sea salt — nothing with added iodine or anti-caking agents, please!

We use a base recipe of 200 g (7 oz) salt to 3 teaspoons dried spices, seeds or powders, but you can always add more flavouring for a more intense result. Just mix together well, then store in a clean jar or airtight container, in a cool, dry place. Your flavoured salt will keep for up to 1 year, but will be at its best within 6 months, as the flavour will deteriorate over time.

Here are some of our favourite flavour combinations: lime and chilli; lemon and thyme; chilli and cumin; orange and fennel; dill tips, dill seeds and white pepper.

See opposite for tips on drying your herbs, citrus peels and chillies at home.

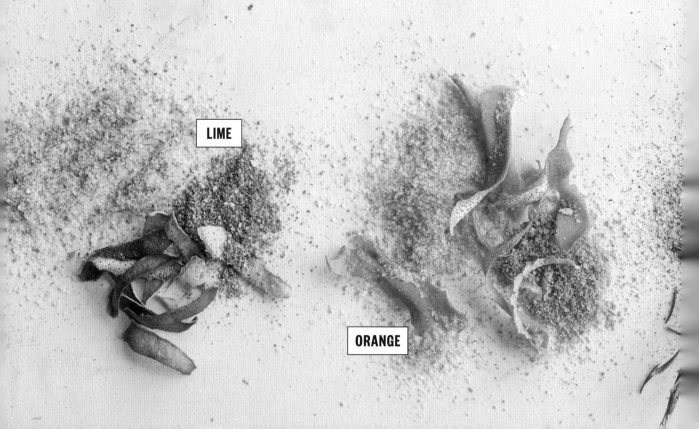

LIME

ORANGE

DRYING HERBS

Tie fresh herbs such as rosemary, thyme, oregano, dill, sage and curry leaves in small bundles and hang upside down in a dry warm spot. We often hang them in the kitchen window, out of direct sunlight. When the herbs are completely dry, which we find usually takes 2–4 days, strip the leaves off the stems and store in airtight containers.

If you want to dry fresh herbs quickly, spread the herbs on a baking tray and leave in a preheated 140°C (285°F) oven until the herbs are completely dry. Woody herbs such as rosemary and thyme will only take about 10–15 minutes, whereas softer herbs such as mint and dill will take a lot longer. When cool and completely dry, crush the coarser herbs such as dried rosemary, thyme and oregano to a powder, using a mortar and pestle or a spice grinder.

If you're growing your own herbs you can let them go to seed, dry the flowers, then mix them through your salts. We do this with the fennel that grows wild in our neighbourhood.

USING HERB SEEDS

To use seeds such as fennel, coriander, cumin and celery seeds, just crush them coarsely using a mortar and pestle before adding them to your salt. You can roast them first to intensify the flavour.

DRYING CITRUS PEELS

Peel your chosen variety of citrus into thin strips, avoiding as much of the bitter white pith as you can. Spread the strips on a baking tray and leave in a preheated 140°C (285°F) oven for 15–20 minutes, or until completely dry; it is essential there is no moisture left. Leave to cool, then whiz into a fine powder using a spice grinder. Store in an airtight container.

DRYING CHILLIES

You can buy dried chillies or chilli flakes to make salts, but it is very easy to dry fresh ones. We string up whole chillies on threads and hang them in the window for about a week until dry — but make sure the room is dry and well ventilated, or they will go mouldy.

Alternatively, you can dry them in the oven. Cut the chillies in half lengthways, place on a baking tray lined with baking paper and leave in a preheated 140°C (285°F) oven until completely dry. Depending on the size of the chillies, this can take anywhere between 1 hour and 4 hours. Remove from the oven and leave to cool completely, then place in a spice grinder and mill into flakes or a powder. Store in an airtight container.

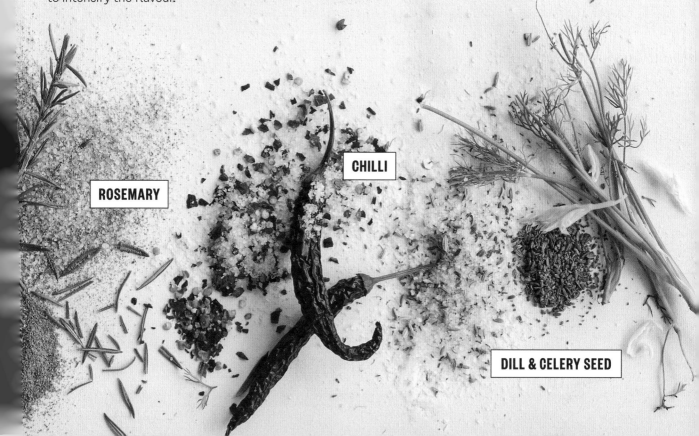

ROSEMARY

CHILLI

DILL & CELERY SEED

PREPARATION TIME	COOKING TIME	SERVES
20 minutes	15 minutes	4

The acidity of the pickled rhubarb adds a refreshing tang to this summer salad. There is no need for a 'proper' dressing — just a splash of lemon juice and olive oil, and maybe a little of the rhubarb pickling liquid.

If you don't have any pickled rhubarb, you could substitute with any other pickle.

CUCUMBER & CELERY SALAD WITH SPROUTS, PICKLED RHUBARB & FRIED HALOUMI

4 Lebanese (short) cucumbers, about 400 g (14 oz) in total
olive oil, for drizzling and pan-frying
2–3 celery stalks, with leaves
250 g (9 oz) haloumi, sliced
3–4 pieces Pickled Rhubarb (page 31), about 50 g (1¾ oz), thinly sliced
1 small handful of sprouts, such as fenugreek, alfalfa or mung bean
1 tablespoon picked oregano or thyme leaves
⅓–½ cup picked dill leaves
juice of 1–2 lemons

Heat a barbecue to medium. Cut two of the cucumbers in half lengthways. Brush them with olive oil, season with salt and pepper and place on the barbecue, cut side down. Char for 5–8 minutes, or until nicely coloured, then set aside to cool.

Slice the remaining cucumbers thinly, using a mandoline or very sharp knife, and place in a large mixing bowl. Thinly slice the celery stalks, reserving the leaves. Chop the charred cucumber into bite-sized pieces and add to the bowl with the celery. Season to taste and set aside.

Heat a good drizzle of olive oil in a frying pan over medium–high heat. Add the haloumi and cook for 2–3 minutes on each side, until golden brown. Drain on paper towel.

Add the reserved celery leaves to the salad, along with the pickled rhubarb, sprouts and three-quarters of the herbs. Lightly toss together.

Place the salad on a large serving plate and arrange the haloumi on top. Squeeze lemon juice over it and drizzle with olive oil, and a dash of the rhubarb pickling juice if desired.

Garnish with the remaining herbs and serve.

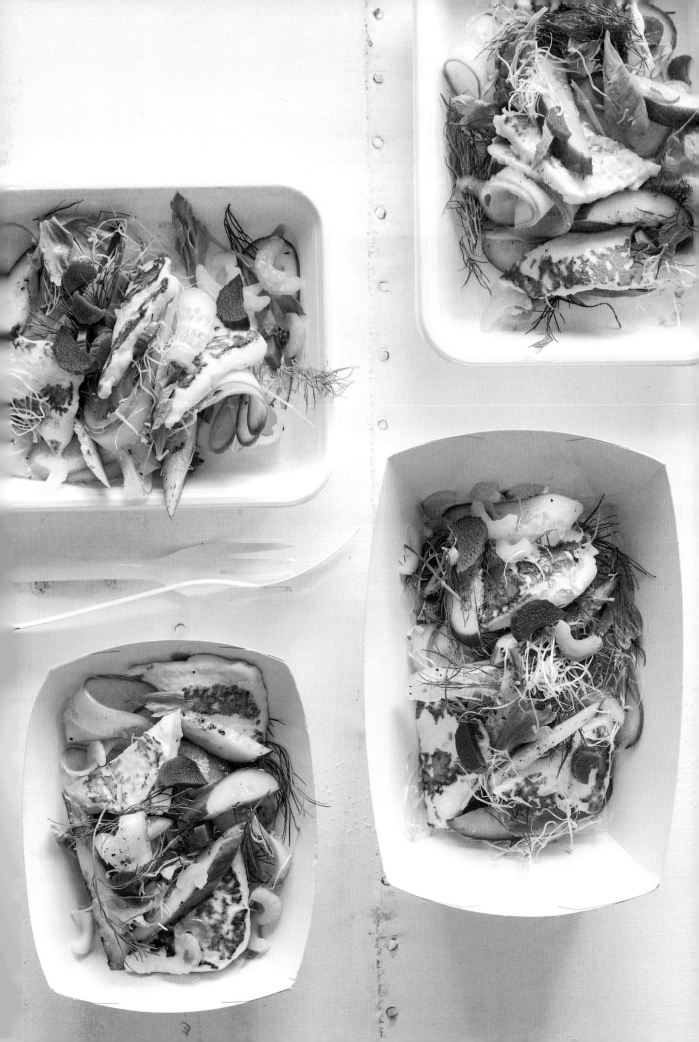

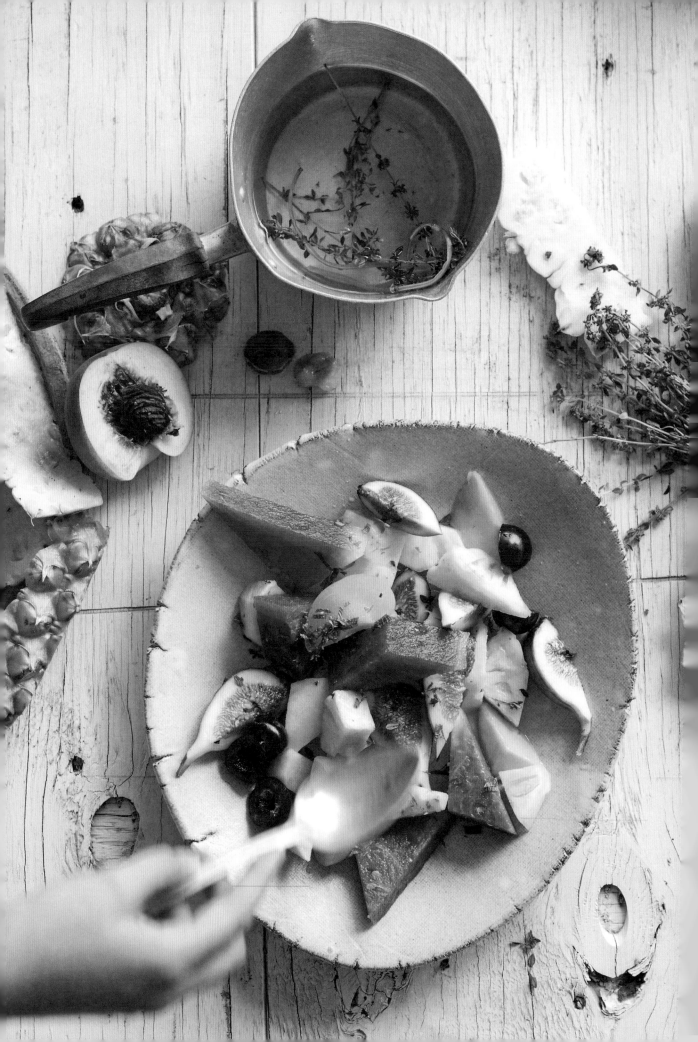

PREPARATION TIME	COOKING TIME	SERVES
15 minutes, plus 30 minutes infusing	10 minutes	4

At Cornersmith we use an abundance of picked herbs, and it seems a shame to throw away the stems that are so full of flavour. Making fragrant syrups is one of the ways we've come up with to reduce our kitchen waste, while at the same time creating something delicious.

In this recipe we use a mint stem syrup to macerate the fruit in. You can also make basil and thyme syrups.

SUMMER FRUIT WITH MINT STEM SYRUP

To make the syrup, put the water and sugar in a small, non-reactive saucepan and bring to a simmer over low heat. Leave to simmer for 5 minutes, then add the mint stems and lemon thyme sprigs and turn off the heat. Let the syrup infuse for about 30 minutes. Stir in the lemon juice and set aside.

Place all the chopped fruit in a large mixing bowl. Add 1–2 tablespoons of the syrup, making sure all the fruit is lightly coated. Adjust the taste to your liking by adding more syrup, or a little more lemon juice. Refrigerate the remaining syrup for another use (see tip).

Place the salad in a serving bowl, or arrange on a platter. Sprinkle the herbs on top and serve immediately — with yoghurt, mascarpone or ice cream, if you're feeling a bit decadent!

TIP: You can make the mint stem syrup in advance, or make a bigger batch and store it in the fridge, where it will keep in a clean airtight container or jar for 1–2 weeks. It is a lovely addition to mineral water as an alternative to cordial, in an alcoholic spritz, or mixed through lemonade with some citrus and cucumber.

1 mango, flesh cut into bite-sized pieces
250 g (9 oz) chunk of watermelon, rind removed (see page 90), cut into bite-sized pieces
300 g (10½ oz) chunk of pineapple, skin and core removed, cut into bite-sized pieces
1 handful of cherries, pitted and cut in half
2 figs, cut lengthways into quarters
2 summer stone fruit, such as peaches, nectarines or apricots, pitted and cut into quarters or bite-sized pieces
1 teaspoon picked lemon thyme leaves
1 teaspoon thinly sliced mint leaves

MINT STEM SYRUP
300 ml (10½ fl oz) water
150 g (5½ oz) sugar
2 mint stems, broken into pieces to release the aroma
2 lemon thyme sprigs
juice of 1 lemon

PREPARATION TIME	FERMENTING TIME	STORAGE	MAKES
15 minutes, plus 2 hours saltings, plus 20 minutes sterilising	at least 2 days	6 months	2–3 x 500 ml (17 fl oz/2 cup) jars

These are a staple pickle on Eastern European tables. At Cornersmith we love to eat them over spring and summer. They're great on a cheese plate, or sliced in a salad, and have even been described as vegan 'salami'! You can use completely green tomatoes, or under-ripe tomatoes that are just starting to turn red.

This version, by our resident fermenter Jaimee Edwards, was inspired by a recipe from one of her food heroes, Ukrainian chef and food writer Olia Hercules.

FERMENTED TOMATOES WITH CELERY & CARAWAY

1 kg (2 lb 4 oz) green or
    under-ripe tomatoes,
    quartered
200 g (7 oz) celery stalks
    and leaves, chopped
2 teaspoons caraway seeds
2 teaspoons black peppercorns
2 teaspoons sea salt

Toss all the ingredients together in a mixing bowl. Set aside for at least 1–2 hours to draw the moisture from the tomatoes.

Sterilise your jars and lids (see page 212).

Pack the mixture into the jars, including the salty liquid that has released from the tomatoes, pressing down as you pack to release more liquid.

Once packed, the tomatoes need to be covered by about 1 cm (½ inch) of liquid; if they aren't, simply top up the jars with water.

Seal the lids, then place your jars out of direct sunlight for 2–7 days, depending on how warm the ambient temperature is. The warmer the weather, the faster your vegetables will ferment.

Open your jar every few days to 'burp' your ferment — this will release the built-up carbon dioxide, and prevent brine spilling out of the jar. Just be sure to press down your mixture afterwards, so that the brine is covering the top by at least 1 cm (½ inch). If any brine does escape, simply wipe the jar down.

After 2 days, taste your tomatoes. If you like them, place them in the fridge, where they will last for up to 6 months.

If you want to ferment your tomatoes further, keep checking and tasting every 2 days until you are happy with the flavour, then store in the fridge.

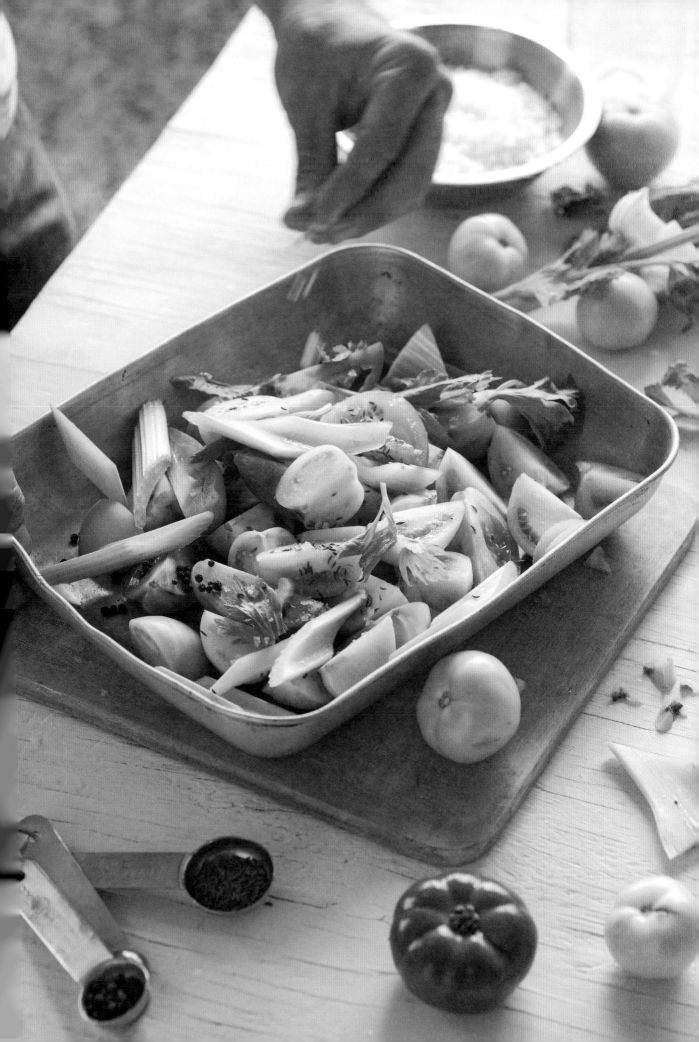

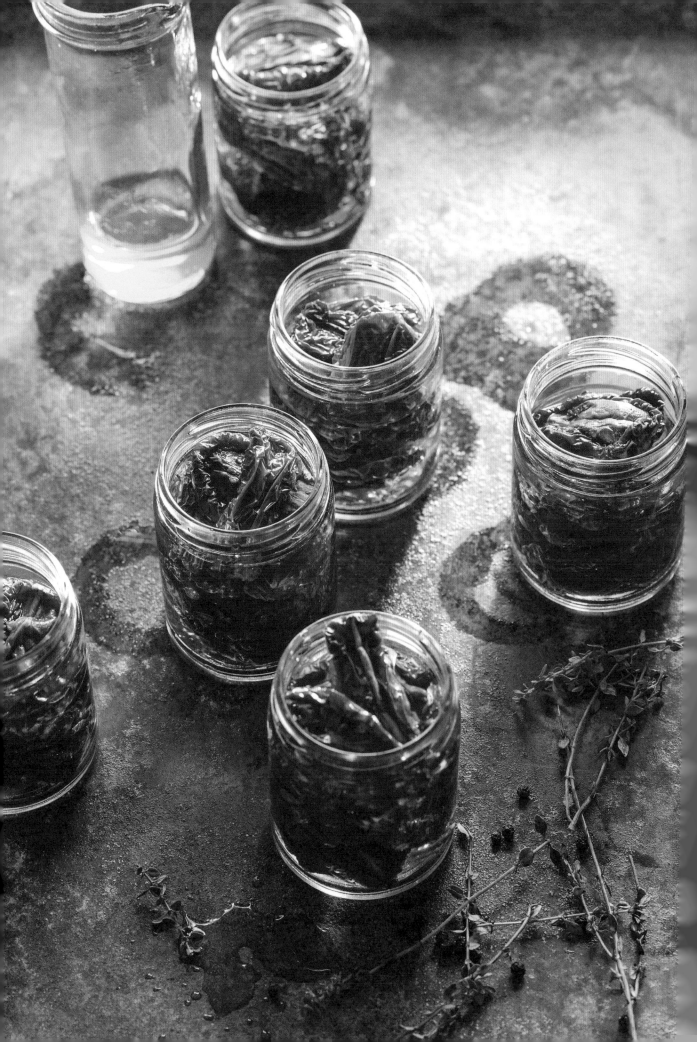

PREPARATION TIME	COOKING TIME	STORAGE	MAKES
20 minutes, plus 20 minutes sterilising	10 minutes, plus at least 7 hours drying	up to 6 months	3 x 300 ml (10½ fl oz) jars

This is a great recipe when you're completely overloaded with tomatoes. These preserved tomatoes are so full of flavour and are excellent thinly sliced through pasta, in tomato salads, or with ricotta and lots of pepper on toast.

OVEN-DRIED PRESERVED TOMATOES

Preheat your oven to its lowest setting. We set ours to 65°C (150°F), but most domestic ovens can only go as low as 100°C (210°F). You can also use a dehydrator if you have one.

Wash your tomatoes and cut them in halves or quarters, depending on their size. Place on a baking tray lined with baking paper, or on a wire rack set over a baking tray. Sprinkle with the salt and place in the oven.

For ovens set to 100°C (210°F), the tomatoes can take 7–9 hours to dry. For ovens set to 65°C (150°F), the tomatoes can take 10–12 hours to dry. You want your tomatoes to be mostly dried, but still maintain some plumpness. If your oven feels too hot, you can wedge the door open with a wooden spoon to increase the airflow. (If using a dehydrator, refer to the manufacturer's instructions for advice on a suitable length of drying time.)

When the tomatoes have finished drying, leave to cool completely.

Sterilise your jars and lids (see page 212).

Make your brine by combining the vinegar, water and sugar in a small, non-reactive saucepan. Place over low heat and stir to dissolve the sugar. Bring to simmering point, then turn off the heat.

When the jars are cool enough to handle, add any spices or herbs you wish to use, such as 1 garlic clove, 4 peppercorns and 1 thyme sprig. Using small clean tongs or clean hands, carefully pack the dried tomatoes into the jars. Pour the hot brine over the tomatoes, filling each jar only three-quarters of the way up.

Remove any air bubbles by gently tapping each jar on the work surface and sliding a clean butter knife or chopstick around the inside of the jars to release any hidden air pockets. Fill each jar with oil, leaving a 5 mm (¼ inch) gap at the top. Wipe the rims of the jars with paper towel or a clean damp cloth and seal immediately.

Leave to cool on the benchtop, then store in a cool, dark place for up to 6 months. If the weather is particularly hot, store the tomatoes in the fridge.

Once opened, refrigerate and use within 3 months.

2 kg (4 lb 8 oz) tomatoes
2 teaspoons salt
375 ml (13 fl oz/1½ cups) white wine vinegar
185 ml (6 fl oz/¾ cup) water
75 g (2½ oz/⅓ cup) sugar
optional flavourings, such as peeled garlic, black peppercorns, thyme, oregano sprigs and/or basil stems
150–200 ml (5–7 fl oz) olive oil or vegetable oil

PREPARATION TIME	COOKING TIME	SERVES
20 minutes, plus 15 minutes resting	15 minutes	4

This salad features heavily in our obsessive fig-eating mission over the summer months. It works as a light summer meal on its own, or as a side dish.

Pearl couscous, also known as Israeli couscous, has a nuttier flavour and more pronounced texture than regular couscous, its much smaller cousin.

Za'atar is a fragrant Middle Eastern spice mix based on dried thyme and sumac. Its 'zing' and freshness complement the sweetness of the figs really well. You'll find it in Middle Eastern grocery stores, spice shops and well-stocked supermarkets — or you could experiment with making your own.

FIG & HERB SALAD WITH PEARL COUSCOUS, TOASTED HAZELNUTS & ZA'ATAR

200 g (7 oz) pearl couscous
6–8 figs, depending on their size
2 tablespoons olive oil, plus extra for drizzling
1½ tablespoons sherry vinegar
1 small handful of picked chervil and/or oregano leaves
1 small handful of picked flat-leaf (Italian) parsley leaves
1 small handful of picked basil leaves
1 teaspoon picked thyme leaves
45 g (1½ oz/⅓ cup) toasted hazelnuts (see page 206), roughly chopped
½ teaspoon za'atar
dried pollen from 2–3 fennel flower heads (optional; see tip)

Bring 500 ml (17 fl oz/2 cups) water to the boil in a saucepan over medium heat. Add some salt and stir in the couscous. Reduce the heat and let the couscous simmer just below boiling point for 5–10 minutes, or until it has absorbed the liquid and is firm but tender, stirring every minute or so. Turn off the heat and cover the pan with a lid. Leave to steam for 10–15 minutes, then loosen the couscous with a fork and set aside to cool.

Meanwhile, prepare the figs. Cut off the stems, then tear the figs into bite-sized pieces. Place in a mixing bowl, season with salt and pepper, drizzle with the oil and vinegar and let them macerate for about 5 minutes.

Gently fold most of the herbs and most of the hazelnuts through the figs, being careful not to break them up too much.

Spread the couscous on a large serving plate or platter. Arrange the figs and herbs on top. Garnish with the remaining herbs and nuts and sprinkle the za'atar evenly over the salad. Finish with an extra drizzle of olive oil, crumble the fennel pollen on top, if using, and serve.

TIP: You'll often find fennel growing wild along roadsides and railway lines. Pick the flower heads, then hang them upside down in a well-ventilated spot in your kitchen for 2–3 days, until dry. Crumble the dried fennel pollen over dishes, or use the pollen or flowers to infuse honey or vinegar, or to flavour your pickles.

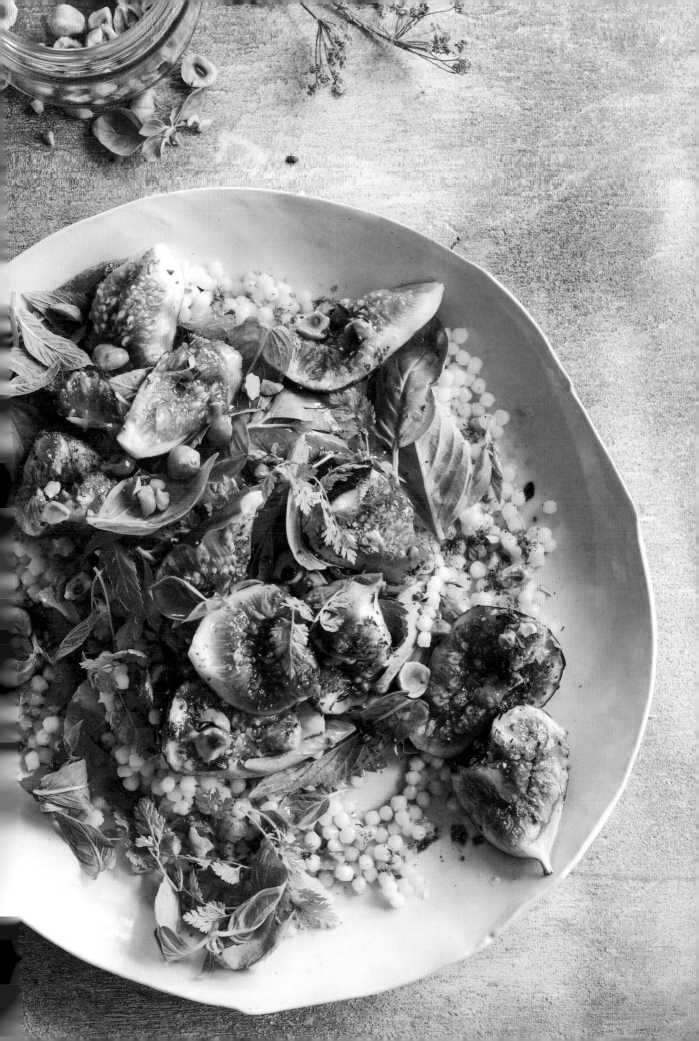

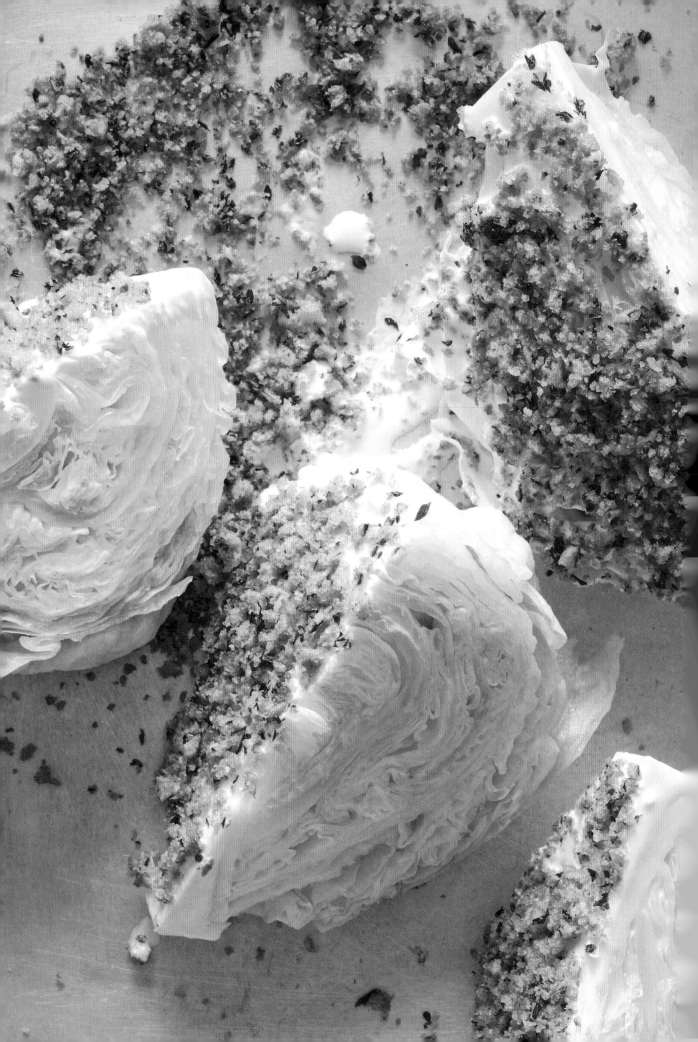

These lettuce wedges are a great addition to a summer barbecue. Fresh, crispy and full of flavour, they are also an excellent way to use up stale bread. Don't drown the wedges in too much dressing — you want lightness and crunch.

ICEBERG WEDGES WITH AIOLI YOGHURT SAUCE & HERB CRUST

To make the aioli, place the egg yolks, vinegar, mustard, garlic and salt in a food processor or blender. Start the machine and add the vegetable oil in a thin, steady stream — be sure to do this really slowly, or the aioli may split. Blend until the mixture is thick and creamy, then taste and add a pinch of salt if needed.

To make the breadcrumb crust, place the bread, herbs and garlic in a food processor and blend into fine crumbs.

Heat the olive oil in a large frying pan over medium heat. Add the breadcrumb mixture and fry, stirring constantly, for 3–5 minutes, until the crumbs are golden brown and crispy in texture. Season with salt and pepper, tip into a big bowl and leave to cool.

Meanwhile, in a small bowl, mix together the yoghurt and 2 tablespoons of the aioli, keep the remaining aioli in a clean airtight container in the fridge for later use (see tip). Check the seasoning, but don't oversalt the yoghurt sauce, as the breadcrumb crust is seasoned as well.

Place the lettuce wedges on serving plates. Spread one-quarter of the aioli yoghurt sauce over one cut side of each lettuce wedge. Cover with the breadcrumb crust, so it sticks to the sauce. Any leftover crust mixture will keep for 3–4 days in an airtight container for sprinkling over other dishes.

Serve immediately.

1 iceberg lettuce, about 400 g (14 oz), outer leaves removed, cut lengthways into quarters
2 tablespoons natural unsweetened yoghurt

FOR THE AIOLI
2 free-range egg yolks
1½ teaspoons white wine vinegar
1 teaspoon dijon mustard
1 garlic clove, crushed
pinch of sea salt
260 ml (9¼ fl oz) vegetable oil

FOR THE BREADCRUMB CRUST
100 g (3½ oz) stale bread, crust removed, cut into little cubes
1 small handful of picked parsley leaves
1 teaspoon picked thyme leaves
1 garlic clove, roughly chopped
1½ tablespoons olive oil

TIP: When making the aioli, reserve the egg whites for recipes such as the salted almonds in the pickled stone fruit salad on page 94. Of course you can use bought mayonnaise here, but home-made aioli tastes so much better, and is a beautiful rich sauce to have on hand for the summer barbecue dishes such as the Whole Grilled Corn on page 64. Any leftovers will keep in the fridge for 3–4 days, and you can add all kinds of flavours, such as finely chopped preserved lemon rind, pickled gherkins and/or capers, or a few teaspoons of blood orange juice.

PREPARATION TIME	COOKING TIME	STORAGE	MAKES
30 minutes, plus 20 minutes sterilising, plus 10 minutes heat-processing (optional)	about 1¼ hours	6 months, or up to 2 years if heat-processed	4 x 300 ml (10½ fl oz) jars

A Cornersmith favourite! We can't make enough of this relish to keep our customers happy, so here's the recipe. It's great at barbecues, with potatoes and polenta; also try it with the Potato & Roasted Chickpea Salad on page 182.

RED PEPPER RELISH

170 ml (5½ fl oz/⅔ cup) olive or vegetable oil
500 g (1 lb 2 oz) onions, thinly sliced
1.5 kg (3 lb 5 oz) red capsicums (peppers), cut into long strips 1–2 cm (½ inch) thick
2–3 garlic cloves, crushed or finely chopped
1–2 teaspoons smoked paprika
2 teaspoons ground cumin
1 teaspoon ground caraway seeds
½ teaspoon chilli flakes
500 ml (17 fl oz/2 cups) red wine vinegar
110 g (3¾ oz/½ cup) caster (superfine) sugar
2 teaspoons salt

Heat the oil in a non-reactive saucepan over medium heat. Add half the onion and sauté for about 10 minutes, or until starting to soften. Add the remaining onion and sauté for another 5 minutes or so.

Add half the capsicum and cook out any liquid that is released, then add the remaining capsicum and turn up the heat. Stir constantly to soften the vegetables, making sure the excess liquid evaporates and the vegetables aren't stewing in their own juices. This will take around 15–20 minutes.

Once the capsicum is soft but not falling apart, add the garlic and sauté until fragrant. Add the spices and mix well.

Now add the vinegar, sugar and salt, stirring until the sugar and salt have dissolved. Turn the heat down to low and cook gently for about 45 minutes, or until the relish is starting to thicken. Turn up the heat for the last 5 minutes and cook out any excess liquid.

Meanwhile, sterilise your jars and lids (see page 212).

Carefully fill the hot jars with the hot relish. Remove any air bubbles by gently tapping each jar on the work surface and sliding a clean butter knife around the inside to release any hidden air pockets. Wipe the rims of the jars with paper towel or a clean damp cloth and seal immediately.

Store in a cool, dark place for up to 6 months. To extend the shelf life to 2 years, heat-process the jars (see page 211) for 10 minutes.

Leave to sit for at least 1 month before eating. Once opened, refrigerate and use within 6 months.

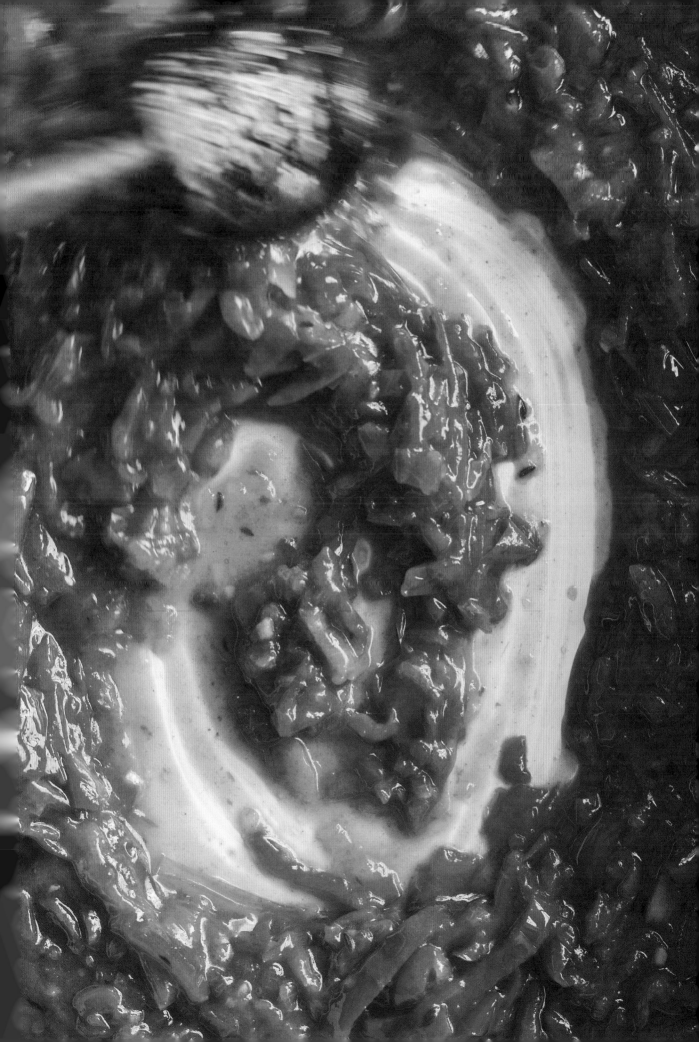

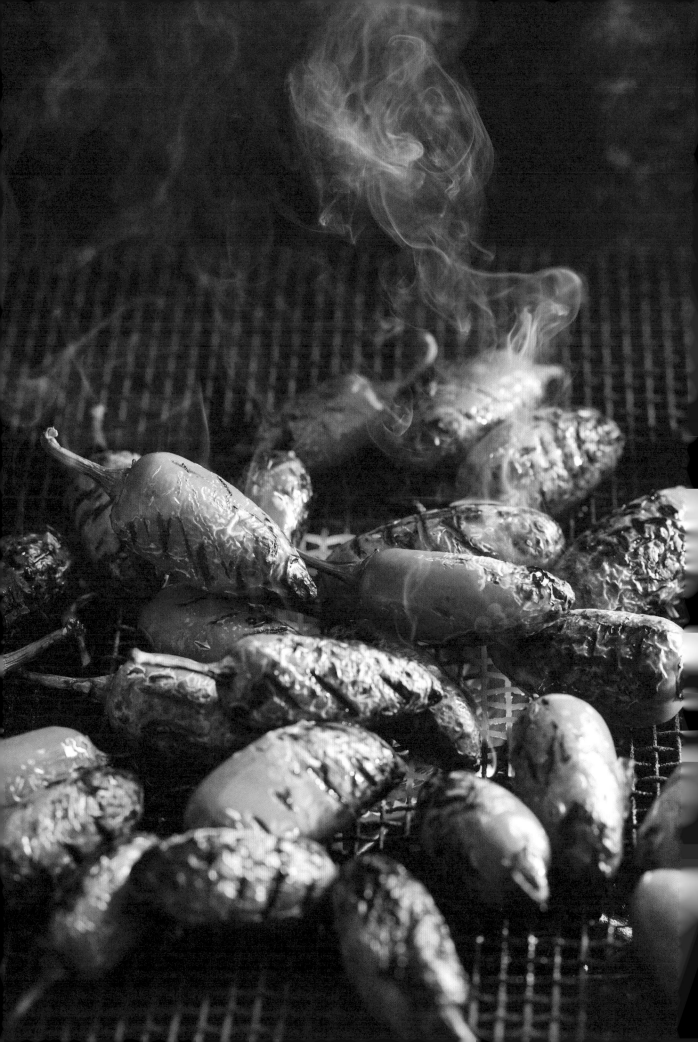

PREPARATION TIME	COOKING TIME	STORAGE	MAKES
25 minutes, plus 20 minutes sterilising, plus 15 minutes heat processing	20 minutes	up to 2 years	2 x 500 ml (17 fl oz) jars

If you're into chillies, make a few jars of these. You can pickle them raw, or lightly char or smoke them for added flavour and sweetness. We don't generally use spices in this recipe — it's more about preserving the jalapeños when the season is in full swing, to use later in the year. However, you could add a slice of ginger, a few black peppercorns, some mustard seeds and a garlic clove to each jar.

You can serve these straight out of the jar, on tacos or burgers. To make a quick, simple salsa, roughly chop a few charred pickled jalapeños with fresh coriander (cilantro) and red onion, then season with salt and pepper.

PICKLED CHARRED JALAPEÑOS

Lightly char the whole chillies, without using any oil. The easiest way to do this is on a barbecue, chargrill pan or over a gas flame; this will usually take about 10–15 minutes. Make sure you turn the chillies regularly, so they are evenly charred and wrinkled all over. (If you have a smoker, even better — the chillies are amazing smoked and then pickled!)

Make your brine by combining the vinegar, water, sugar and salt in a non-reactive, medium-sized saucepan. Place over low heat and stir to dissolve the sugar and salt. Bring to simmering point, then turn off the heat.

Meanwhile, sterilise your jars and lids (see page 212).

When the jars are cool enough to handle, place any spices you may be using in the bottom of each jar. Pack the chillies firmly into the jars, leaving about 1 cm (½ inch) space at the top.

Bring your brine back up to the boil. Pour the hot brine over the chillies, making sure they are completely submerged. You may need to pack in more chillies once they've softened in the hot brine. The more tightly packed the jars are, the less chance there is of the chillies floating and not preserving properly.

Remove any air bubbles by gently tapping each jar on the work surface and sliding a clean butter knife or chopstick around the inside to release any hidden air pockets. Wipe the rims of the jars with paper towel or a clean damp cloth and seal.

Heat-process (see page 211) for 15 minutes, then store in a cool, dark place for up to 2 years.

Once opened, refrigerate and use within 6 months.

500 g (1 lb 2 oz) jalapeño chillies (or any chillies of your choice), pierced with a sharp knife to allow the vinegar to seep in during pickling
350 ml (12 fl oz) white wine vinegar
170 ml (5½ fl oz/⅔ cup) water
45 g (1½ oz/scant ¼ cup) sugar
1½ teaspoons salt

PREPARATION TIME	STORAGE	MAKES
20 minutes, plus overnight salting	up to 2 months	1 x 750 ml (26 fl oz) jar or container

This is a great recipe to use up the rind from all the watermelon that gets eaten over summer. We toss this pickle through our Watermelon & Feta Salad on page 93, but it is also delicious on a cheese plate, or added to other salads.

You can heat-process this pickle to make it last longer, but the texture will be better if you store it in the fridge.

PICKLED WATERMELON RIND

250 g (9 oz) peeled watermelon
    rind
3 tablespoons salt

FOR THE BRINE
400 ml (14 fl oz) apple cider
    vinegar
200 ml (7 fl oz) water
165 g (5¾ oz/¾ cup) sugar
1 tablespoon salt
4 slices fresh ginger
½ teaspoon chilli flakes
1 teaspoon allspice berries
3–4 juniper berries
2 star anise
1 teaspoon black peppercorns

Peel off and discard the green outer skin from the watermelon rind.

Slice the white flesh of the watermelon rind into strips and place in a non-reactive container. Sprinkle all over with the salt and leave to stand overnight.

The next day, make your brine by combining all the brine ingredients in a non-reactive, medium-sized saucepan. Place over low heat and stir to dissolve the sugar. Bring to a simmer, then turn off the heat and let the flavours infuse the vinegar for 10 minutes or so.

Rinse the salt off your watermelon rind strips and dry with clean paper towel. Place in a clean container. Cover with the hot spicy brine and allow to cool.

Once cool, cover with a lid and store in the fridge. Use within 2 months.

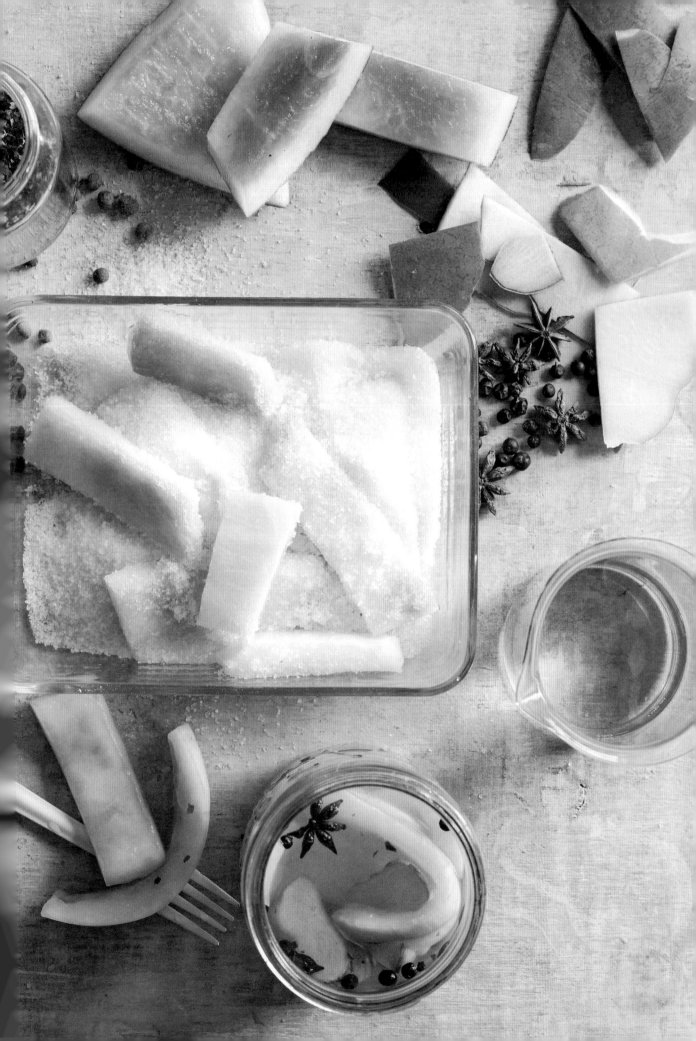

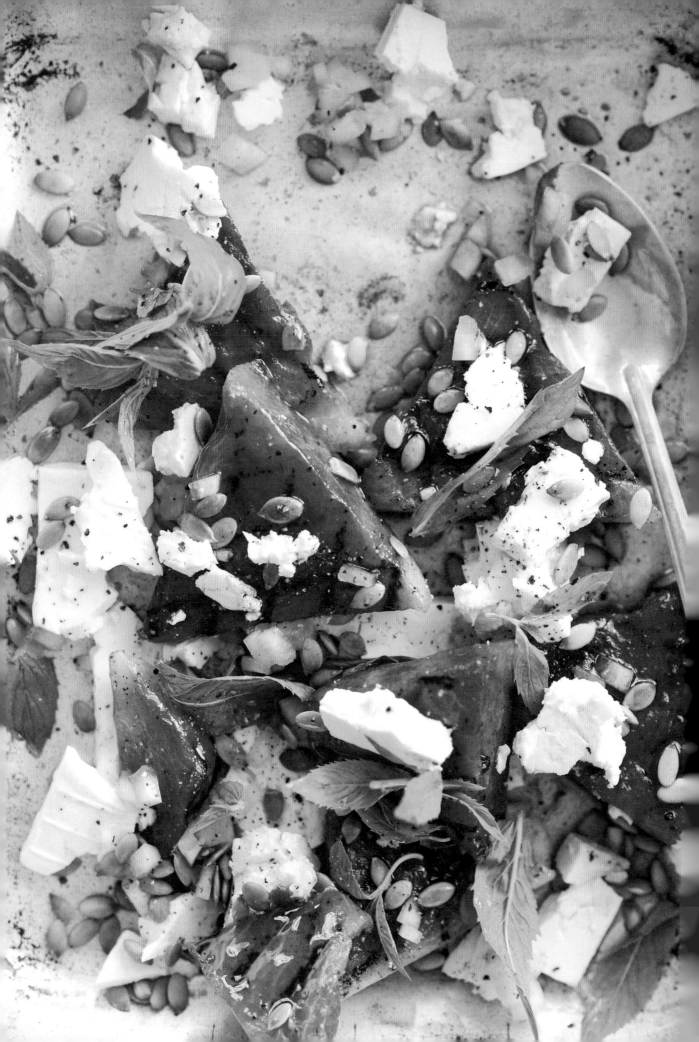

PREPARATION TIME	COOKING TIME	SERVES
15 minutes, plus 30 minutes marinating	10 minutes	4

The inspiration for this refreshing salad comes from a recipe in Peter Gordon's *The Sugar Club Cookbook*, which Sabine first tried back in the late 1990s. It became one of her 'most travelled' recipes, and has delighted people around the world with its simplicity and freshness.

We've added a 'no-waste twist' by pickling leftover watermelon rind. If you don't have the time to marinate and grill the watermelon, or pickle watermelon rind, this salad also works with just fresh watermelon, feta and herbs.

WATERMELON & FETA WITH PICKLED WATERMELON RIND, MINT & PEPITAS

Cut the watermelon flesh into chunky pieces and place in a non-reactive container in a single layer. (They need to be really chunky, so they don't collapse when you grill them on the barbecue.)

Mix together the watermelon pickling juice, olive oil and a sprinkling of salt and pepper. Add the reserved mint stems, torn into pieces. Pour the marinade over the watermelon pieces, keeping them in a single layer. Leave to marinate for about 30 minutes.

Heat a barbecue to medium–high. Drain the watermelon chunks well, reserving the marinade. Quickly sear them on the barbecue for just 1–2 minutes on each side – you don't want them to collapse and lose all their juiciness.

Transfer the watermelon to a serving plate. Arrange the feta and pickled watermelon rind around. Strain the reserved marinating liquid and drizzle 1–2 tablespoons over the salad. Season with pepper and drizzle with a little extra olive oil.

Sprinkle with lemon juice to taste, and a little salt if you think it needs it, remembering that feta is very salty. Finish off with the mint leaves and pepitas and serve.

750 g (1 lb 10 oz) watermelon flesh, rind removed (see tip)
2 tablespoons finely diced Pickled watermelon rind (page 90), plus about 100 ml (3½ fl oz) of the pickling juice
2 tablespoons olive oil, plus extra for drizzling over the salad
1 handful of picked mint leaves; reserve the mint stems for the marinade
200–250 g (7–9 oz) feta cheese, sliced or broken into bite-sized chunks
juice of ½–1 lemon
2 tablespoons toasted pepitas (pumpkin seeds); see page 206

TIP: Reserve the watermelon rind and pickle it using the recipe on page 90. If you'd like to add a bit more 'body' to the salad, toss through some peppery rocket (arugula) leaves.

PREPARATION TIME	COOKING TIME	SERVES
20 minutes	15 minutes	4

This quick, summery salad is simple, light and delicious. If you don't have pickled stone fruit, you could grill or roast some peaches or plums instead.

The salted almonds make a great snack, so make a larger batch and keep them in an airtight container. They're a perfect way to use up leftover egg whites. Try spicing them up with a pinch of smoked paprika or cumin.

SUMMER LEAVES, PICKLED STONE FRUIT, RICOTTA & SALTED ALMONDS

4–6 Pickled Peach halves (page 97), plus 1 tablespoon of the pickling liquid
100 g (3½ oz) bunch of rocket (arugula)
6–8 baby cos (romaine) lettuce leaves, or 1 small cos lettuce
2 teaspoons balsamic vinegar
2½ tablespoons olive oil
125 g (4½ oz) fresh ricotta cheese

SALTED ALMONDS
1 free-range egg white
1–2 pinches of sea salt
60 g (2¼ oz/heaped ⅓ cup) blanched almonds

Preheat the oven to 150–160°C (300–315°F). Line a baking tray with baking paper.

To make the salted almonds, place the egg white in a bowl and beat lightly with a fork or small whisk until it becomes a bit foamy. Add the salt and beat again to combine. Add the almonds and mix well, to coat them all over with the mixture.

Tip the almonds onto the baking tray and toast in the oven for 8–12 minutes, or until golden brown all over, moving and turning them around on the tray every 3–4 minutes to break up the egg white. Remove from the oven and leave to cool.

Cut the pickled peaches into bite-sized pieces and place in a big mixing bowl. Wash and dry the rocket and lettuce, tear the leaves into pieces, add them to the peaches and gently combine. Season with salt and pepper. Add the pickling liquid, vinegar, olive oil and half the toasted almonds. Mix again gently.

Place the salad on a serving plate or in a bowl. Put dollops of the ricotta on top and sprinkle with the remaining almonds.

Serve the salad immediately.

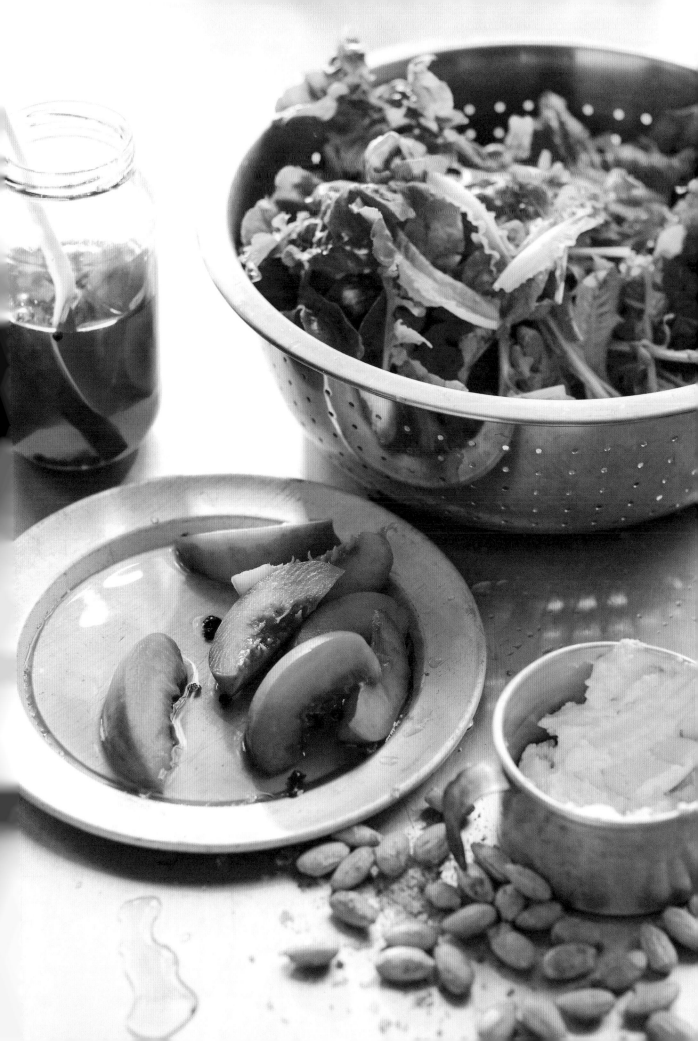

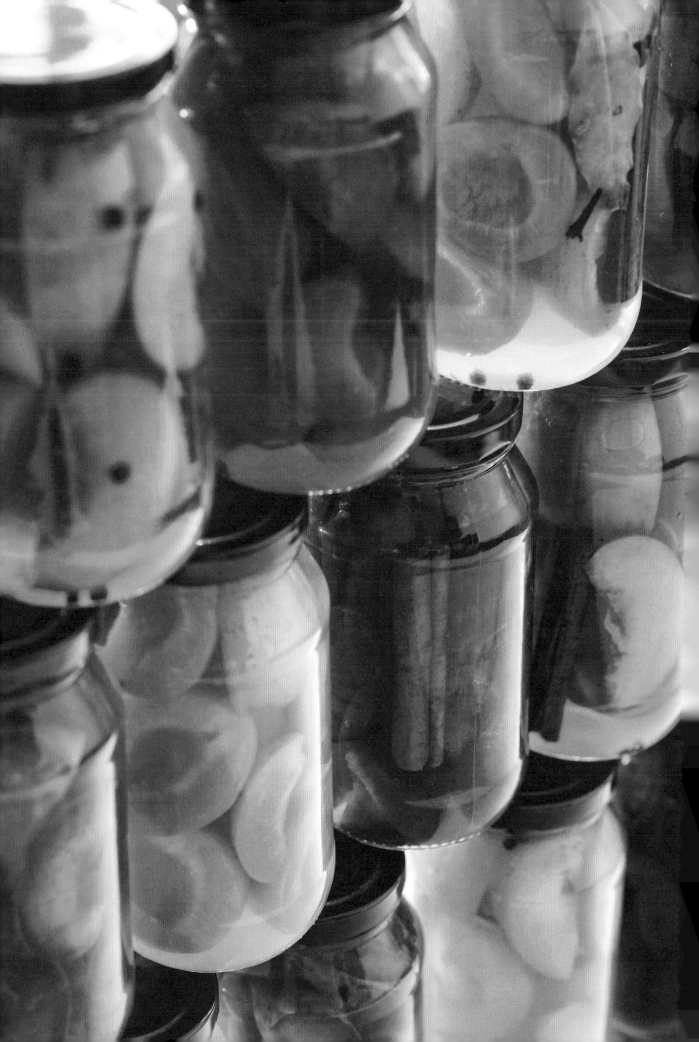

PREPARATION TIME	HEAT-PROCESSING	STORAGE	MAKES
20 minutes, plus 20 minutes sterilising	15 minutes	up to 1 year	3–4 x 500 ml (17 fl oz/2 cup) jars

Pickling is one of our favourite preserving methods for summer fruits. Peaches, nectarines, apricots and plums all work well. Just make sure you use very firm fruit — soft fruit will break down too quickly in the jar.

Experiment with different flavours and combinations — rosemary and peppercorns are great with peaches; ginger and allspice work well with plums.

This brine is sweet and vinegary and makes excellent fruit pickles for a cheese plate, with wintery meats, thinly sliced through a salad, or even served with a dessert. You could also use them in place of any roasted or grilled fruits a recipe calls for. If you're after a more savoury fruit pickle, reduce the sugar by half.

SWEET PICKLED STONE FRUITS

Make your brine by combining the vinegar, water and sugar in a non-reactive, medium-sized saucepan. Place over low heat and stir to dissolve the sugar. Bring to simmering point, then turn off the heat.

Sterilise your jars and lids (see page 212).

When the jars are cool enough to handle, place the spices in the bottom of the jars. Pack the fruit firmly into the hot jars, leaving about 1 cm (½ inch) space at the top.

Bring your brine back up to the boil, then pour the hot brine over the fruit, making sure each piece is completely submerged.

Remove any air bubbles by gently tapping each jar on the work surface and sliding a clean butter knife or chopstick around the inside to release any hidden air pockets. Wipe the rims of the jars with paper towel or a clean damp cloth and seal.

Heat-process (see page 211) for 15 minutes, then store in a cool, dark place for up to 1 year.

Once opened, refrigerate and use within 6 months.

600 ml (21 fl oz) apple cider vinegar
300 ml (10½ fl oz) water
250 g (9 oz) white or raw sugar
1 kg (2 lb 4 oz) firm stone fruit of your choice, cut into quarters or wedges

FOR EACH JAR, YOU WILL NEED:
1 cinnamon stick
4 allspice berries
1 clove
5 black peppercorns

TIP: Save the stones from the stone fruit and make a delicious, fruity almond-flavoured vinegar with them (see page 166). Once you've eaten all your pickles, save the brine! It's great in cocktails, added to salad dressings or drizzled over cakes. Also experiment with other flavours by pickling the stone fruit with other spices of your choice.

PREPARATION TIME	HEAT-PROCESSING	STORAGE	MAKES
20 minutes, plus 20 minutes sterilising	15 minutes	up to 1½ years	2–3 x 500 ml (17 fl oz/2 cup) jars

Sweet pickled cherries are such a treat to have stashed in your pantry. This recipe is nice and easy because you don't even have to pit the cherries!

Try to let these pickles sit for a season or two before you eat them — they get so much better over time, and are amazing with cheese and wine, in cocktails, or sliced through salads.

Once you've eaten all your pickled cherries, don't throw your syrup away! It's great drizzled over fruit with mascarpone, over cakes, or you can reduce it down further and use it as a syrup in soda water or in marinades.

PICKLED CHERRIES

500 ml (17 fl oz/2 cups) red wine vinegar
250 ml (9 fl oz/1 cup) water
250 g (9 oz) raw sugar
8–12 cloves
4–6 star anise
1–1½ teaspoons black peppercorns
1 kg (2 lb 4 oz) cherries

Make your brine by combining the vinegar, water and sugar in a non-reactive, medium-sized saucepan. Place over low heat and stir to dissolve the sugar. Bring to simmering point, then turn off the heat.

Sterilise your jars and lids (see page 212).

When the jars are cool enough to handle, place 4 cloves, 2 star anise and ½ teaspoon peppercorns in the bottom of each jar. Pack the cherries firmly into the hot jars, leaving about 1 cm (½ inch) space at the top.

Bring your brine back up to the boil, then pour the hot brine over the cherries, making sure they are completely submerged. You may need to pack in more cherries once they've softened in the hot brine. The more tightly packed the jars are, the less chance there is of the cherries floating and not preserving properly.

Remove any air bubbles by gently tapping each jar on the work surface and sliding a clean butter knife or chopstick around the inside to release any hidden air pockets. Wipe the rims of the jars with paper towel or a clean damp cloth and seal.

Heat-process (see page 211) for 15 minutes, then store in a cool, dark place for up to 18 months.

Once opened, refrigerate and use within 6 months.

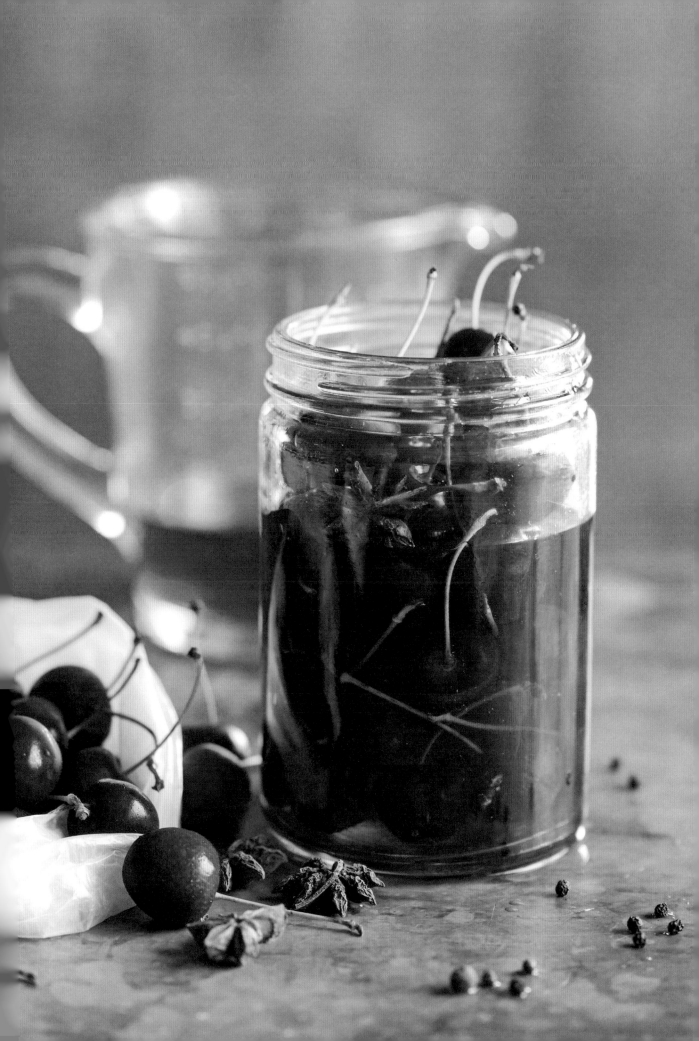

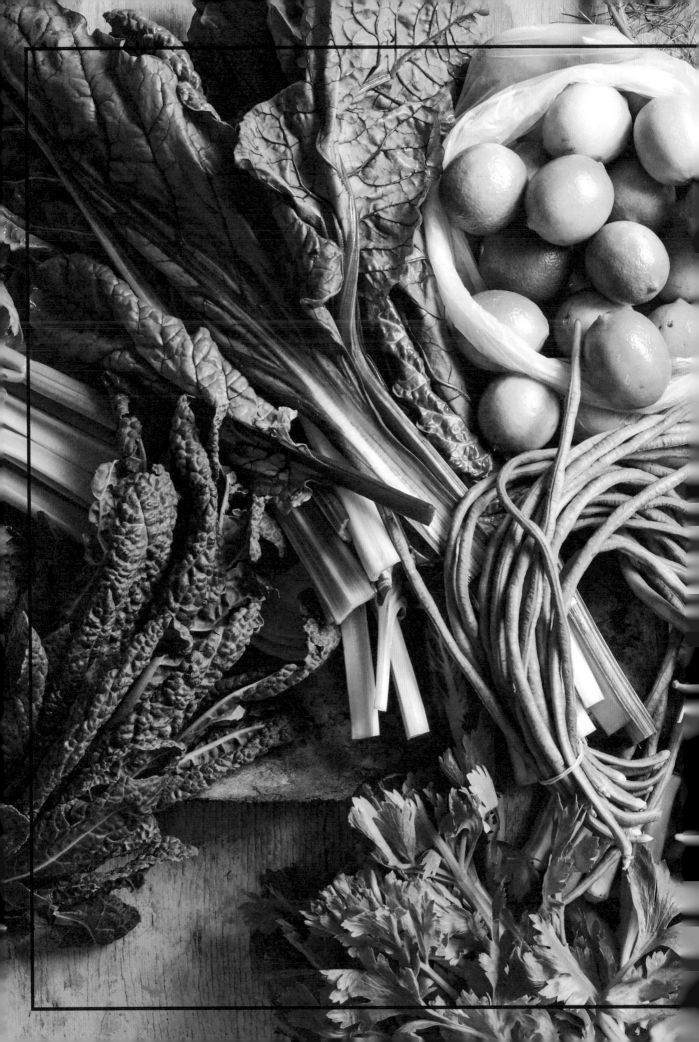

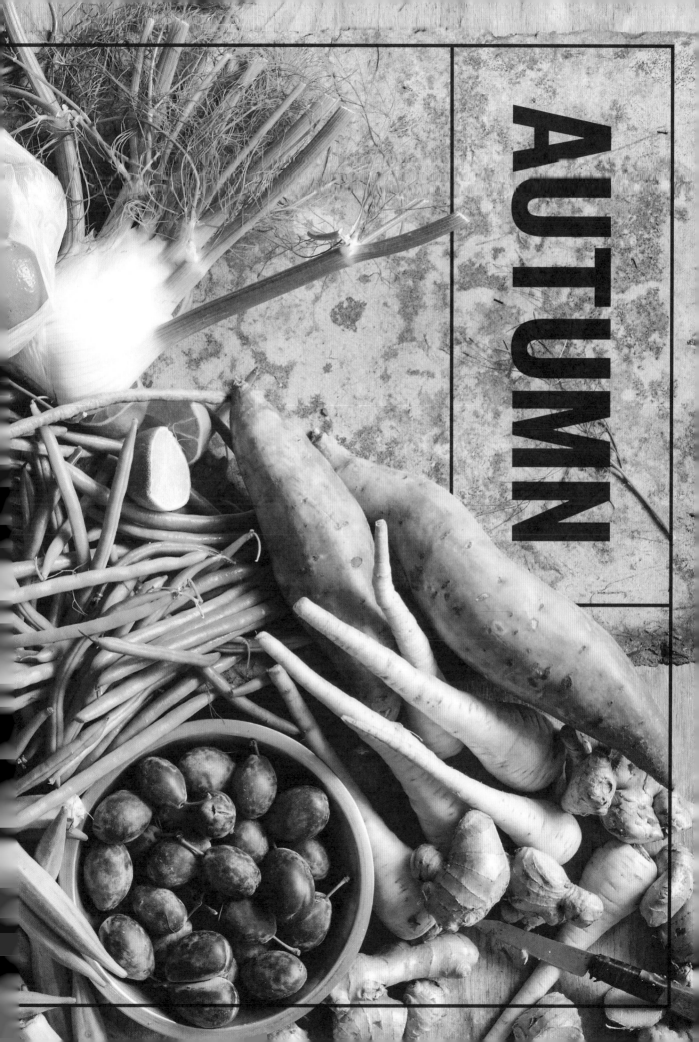

AUTUMN

PREPARATION TIME	SERVES
15 minutes	4

Fresh, tangy and quick to prepare, this slaw often makes an appearance on our autumn menus. It's a great addition to any meal, or to take to a barbecue or picnic, and will easily become part of your salad repertoire.

You can add any other toasted seeds or nuts you have on hand.

AUTUMN SLAW OF CAVOLO NERO, FENNEL & GRAPEFRUIT WITH CHILLI DRESSING

250 g (9 oz) bunch of cavolo nero (black kale)

½ fennel bulb, with fronds

2 pink grapefruit, filleted into segments (see tip)

½ teaspoon finely chopped Salt-Preserved Lemon Skins (see page 187) or preserved lemon rind

1½ tablespoons apple cider vinegar

1 teaspoon Chilli Sambal (page 63)

2 teaspoons citrus marmalade or honey

2–3 tablespoons olive oil

2–3 tablespoons toasted sunflower seeds (see page 206)

Wash the cavolo nero and dry thoroughly. Pluck the leaves off the stems. Very finely chop the stems and place in a large mixing bowl. Tear the leaves into bite-sized pieces, or finely chop them, and add to the bowl.

Thinly slice the fennel bulb, using a mandoline or very sharp knife, and add to the bowl. Finely chop the fennel fronds and set aside.

Add the grapefruit segments and salted lemon skin to the salad and season with salt and pepper.

To make the dressing, combine the vinegar, chilli sambal and marmalade in a screw-top jar. Season with salt and pepper, add the olive oil, put the lid on and shake well to combine. Check the seasoning.

Drizzle the dressing over the salad and combine gently. Transfer to a serving bowl.

Garnish with the reserved fennel fronds and sunflower seeds and serve immediately.

TIP: Keep the grapefruit skins and preserve them in salt (see page 187) to use in your next salad.

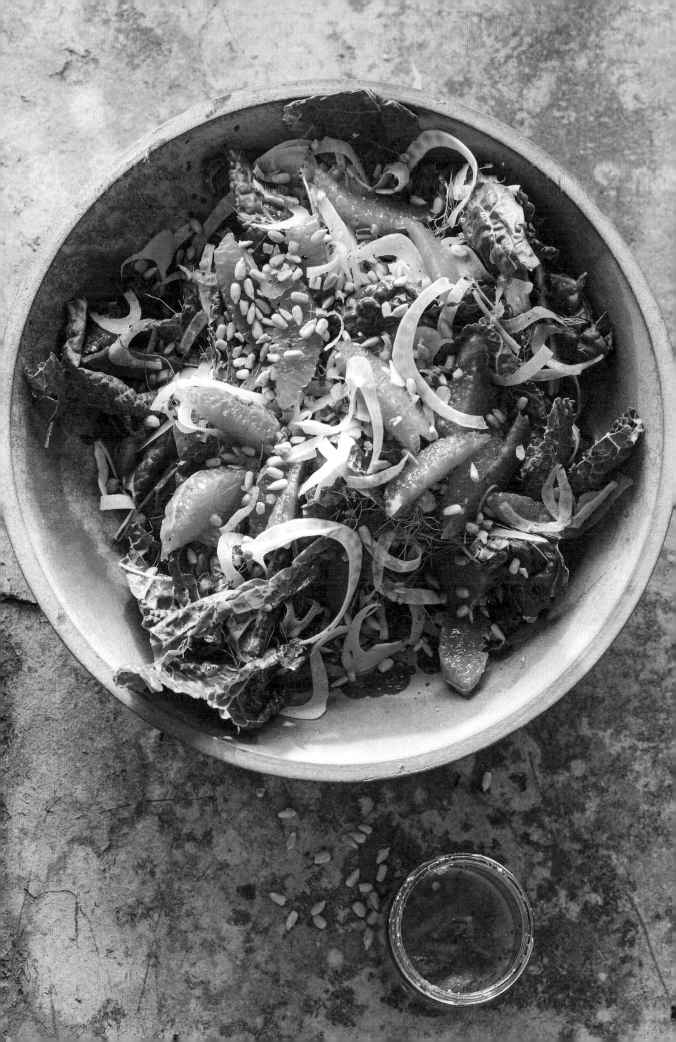

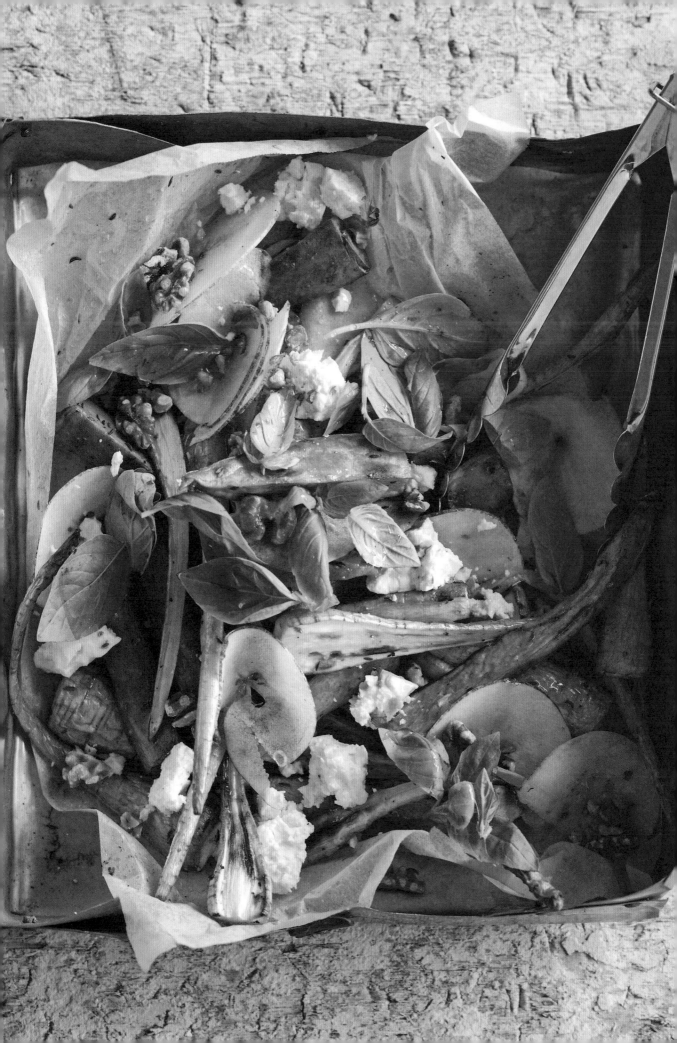

PREPARATION TIME	COOKING TIME	SERVES
25 minutes	20 minutes	4

Some roasted vegie salads can be rather heavy, but here the sweetness of the parsnip and sweet potato is lightened with the fresh acidity of new season apples and the anise notes of basil. If you can't lay your hands on parsnips, you can just replace them with extra sweet potato or carrots.

ROASTED SWEET POTATO & PARSNIP WITH NEW SEASON APPLES, BASIL, WALNUTS & FETA

Preheat the oven to 200°C (400°F). Line a baking tray with baking paper.

Wash the sweet potatoes and parsnips well. Cut the parsnips lengthways into quarters or sixths. Cut the sweet potatoes into wedges about the same size as the parsnips.

Place the parsnip and sweet potato in a large mixing bowl. Add the olive oil, spices, thyme sprigs, garlic cloves and lime zest. Season with salt and pepper and mix well so that the potatoes and parsnips are evenly coated.

Spread the mixture in a single layer on the baking tray. Bake for about 20 minutes, or until golden brown and cooked through.

Transfer to a large mixing bowl and allow the vegetables to cool for a bit.

Cut the apple into quarters and remove the core. Thinly slice, then add to the roasted vegetables with the lime juice, basil and walnuts. Season with salt and pepper and mix gently to combine.

Arrange the salad in a bowl or on a plate. Crumble the feta over and finish with an extra drizzle of olive oil.

Serve warm.

500 g (1 lb 2 oz) sweet potatoes
500 g (1 lb 2 oz) parsnips
2½–3 tablespoons olive oil, plus extra for drizzling over the salad
pinch of cumin seeds
pinch of caraway seeds
pinch of ground cinnamon
1–2 thyme or lemon thyme sprigs
2 garlic cloves, left unpeeled, crushed with the back of a knife
zest and juice of 1–2 limes
1 new season apple
1 handful of picked basil leaves
40 g (1½ oz/⅓ cup) toasted walnuts (see page 206), roughly chopped
80 g (2¾ oz) feta cheese

PREPARATION TIME	COOKING TIME	SERVES
20 minutes	about 1 hour	4

This is a perfect salad for when the weather gets a little cooler. The crusted nashi is so delicious! A firm persimmon would also work well.

Chermoula is a spice paste that makes a great crust on meats and fish, or for roasting vegetables in. It needs to be cooked to soften the raw flavours of the onion, garlic and ginger. You can play around with the heat by adding more or less chilli, fresh or dried, or cayenne pepper; we also use our excess herb stems in it.

CHERMOULA-CRUSTED NASHI PEARS WITH KALE & HAZELNUTS

2 nashi pears
125 ml (4 fl oz/½ cup) water (or half white wine and half water)
1 very ripe tomato, finely chopped
1½ tablespoons olive oil, plus extra for drizzling
2–3 tablespoons (50 g/1¾ oz) toasted hazelnuts (see page 206), roughly crushed
2–3 tablespoons plain yoghurt

CHERMOULA
1 teaspoon cumin seeds
½ teaspoon coriander seeds
½ teaspoon fennel seeds
¼ teaspoon salt
¼ teaspoon ground cinnamon
2 pinches of hot chilli powder
1 cm (½ inch) knob of fresh ginger, peeled and grated
1 garlic clove, peeled
1 small brown onion, chopped
4 kale stems (reserved from below)
45–50 g (1½–1¾ oz) bunch of coriander (cilantro), including the stems
2–2½ tablespoons olive oil

FOR THE KALE
6–7 kale leaves, with stems
½ teaspoon salt
1½ tablespoons apple balsamic vinegar or balsamic vinegar
2 tablespoons hazelnut or olive oil

Preheat the oven to 175°C (350°F).

To make the chermoula, put the cumin, coriander and fennel seeds in a dry frying pan. Toast over medium heat without any oil for 1–2 minutes, until fragrant, stirring so they don't burn. Remove from the heat and leave to cool, then grind to a powder using a spice grinder or mortar and pestle. Add the spices to a food processor, with the salt, cinnamon, chilli powder, ginger, garlic and onion.

Wash the kale stems and finely chop. Pick the coriander leaves off the stems; reserve the leaves for another use. Thoroughly wash and drain the coriander stems and roots, then chop them finely and add to the chermoula with the kale stems. Blend until finely chopped, then add the olive oil and blend to a paste.

Cut the pears in half. Spread the chermoula over the cut side of each pear half. Place the pears, crusted side up, in a baking dish. Add the water and tomato, drizzle with the olive oil and cover the dish with foil. Transfer to the oven and bake for 30–45 minutes.

Remove the foil, turn the oven up to 200°C (400°F) and bake for another 7–10 minutes, until the pears are well crusted, golden brown and just cooked. Set aside to cool, keeping the braising liquid.

Meanwhile, prepare the kale. Cut off the remaining kale stalks and reserve for quick pickling (see page 162). Wash and dry the leaves, tear into smaller pieces and place in a large bowl. Sprinkle with the salt and start 'massaging' the kale leaves with the salt until they start to break down. Season with black pepper, add the vinegar and oil and gently mix to combine.

Place the kale on a large serving plate. Arrange the pears on top of the salad. Sprinkle the hazelnut on top and drizzle with a little extra olive oil, and the yoghurt.

Serve immediately.

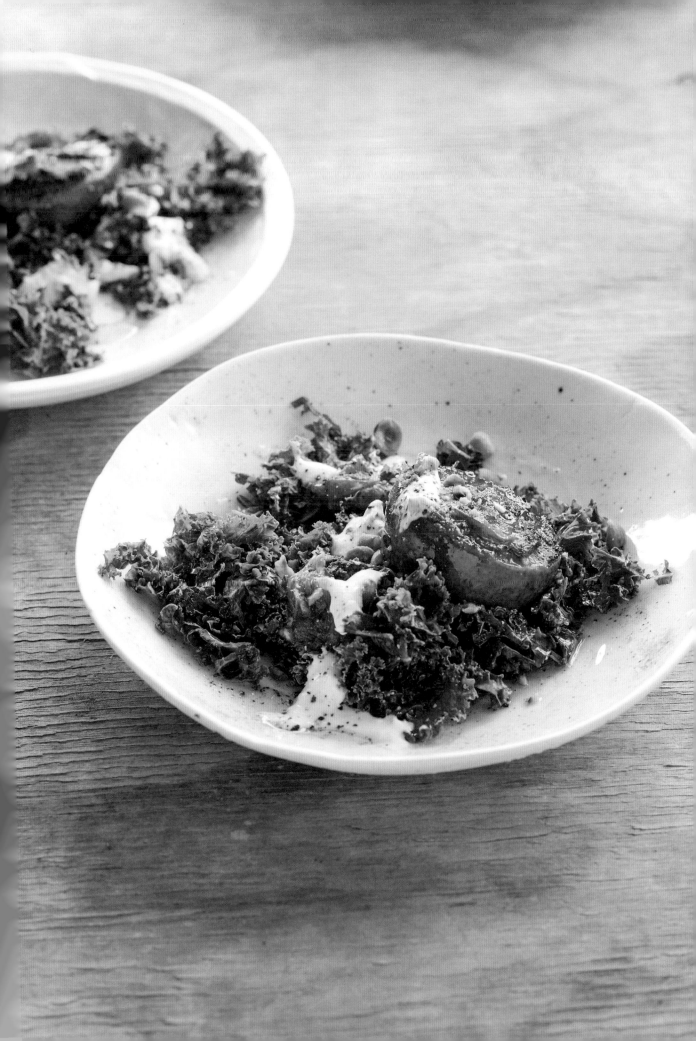

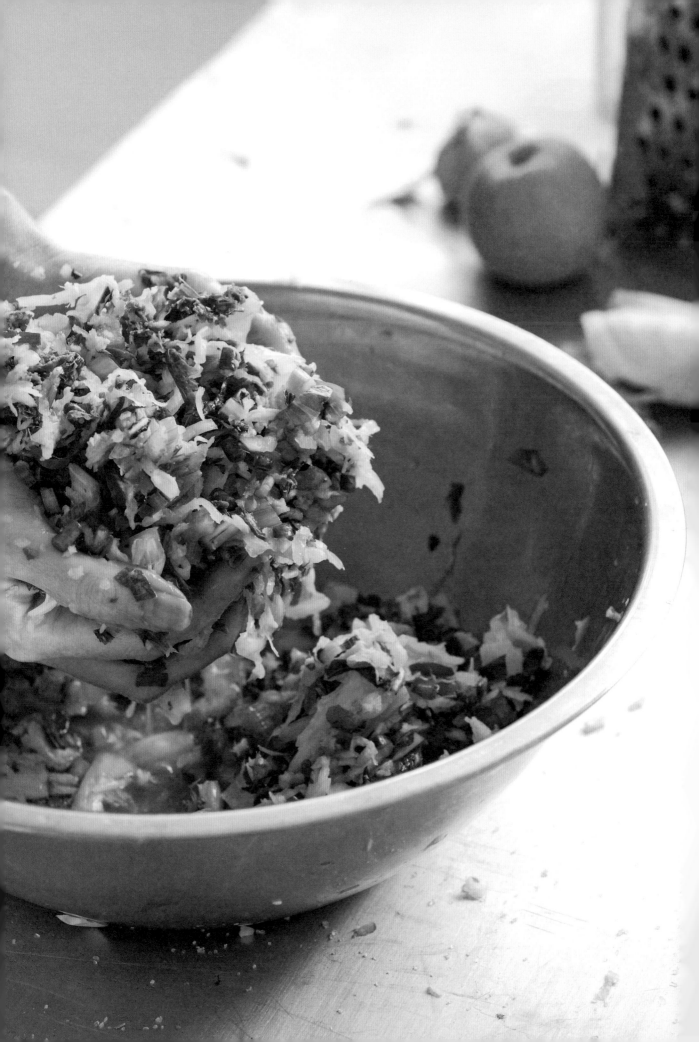

PREPARATION TIME	FERMENTING TIME	STORAGE	MAKES
45 minutes, plus 20 minutes sterilising	2–7 days	6 months	3 x 500 ml (17 fl oz/2 cup) jars

People feel passionately about kimchi, and so they should — it is one of Korea's great culinary gifts to the world. There are many kimchis, from white kimchi to delicate kimchis made with rice water. This recipe is a variation on the more usual red variety, but with a food waste reducing focus. Use up whatever vegetables you have on hand, but keep in mind that a great kimchi balances salty, sour, spicy and a touch of sweet.

KITCHEN SCRAP KIMCHI

Sterilise your jars and lids (see page 212).

Wash all the vegetables. Tear the wombok into large pieces and place in a large mixing bowl.

Peel the daikon, then grate the daikon and ginger into another bowl. Add the garlic, chilli, salt and sugar and mix together. This wet mixture is now your paste.

Prepare whatever other vegetables you are using. Cut them in a uniform way, to the same size. If using pumpkin, cut it into thin matchsticks, including the skin.

Add these vegetables to your wombok and gently massage together until all the water is released. Once your vegetables feel wet, add your daikon paste and keep massaging. You want to be able to pick up a handful of vegetables and see water running when you give them a gentle squeeze.

Once this happens, pack your vegetables into your cooled, sterilised jars, pressing down to release air bubbles as you go, and leaving 2 cm (¾ inch) clear space at the top of the jars. The surface of your vegetables should be covered with 1 cm (½ inch) of liquid. If not, simply top up with water. Wipe the rim of the jars with paper towel or a clean damp cloth and seal.

Place your jars out of direct sunlight for 2–7 days, depending on how warm the ambient temperature is. The warmer the weather, the faster your vegetables will ferment. Open your jar every few days to 'burp' your ferment — this will release the built-up carbon dioxide, and prevent brine spilling out of the jar. Just be sure to press down your kimchi afterwards, so that the brine is covering the top by at least 1 cm (½ inch). If any brine does escape, simply wipe the jar down.

After 2 days, taste your kimchi. If you like it, place it in the refrigerator, where it will last for up to 6 months.

If you want to ferment your kimchi further, keep checking and tasting every 2 days until you are happy with the flavour, then store in the fridge.

500 g (1 lb 2 oz) wombok (Chinese cabbage)
500 g (1 lb 2 oz) daikon
750 g (1 lb 10 oz) mixed vegetables and fruit, such as pumpkin (winter squash), carrots, kale and kale stems, chokos (chayote), nashi pears and radish tops
100 g (3½ oz) fresh ginger
4 garlic cloves, crushed
1 tablespoon chilli flakes
1¼ tablespoons salt
½ teaspoon sugar

PREPARATION TIME	STORAGE	MAKES
30 minutes, plus 20 minutes sterilising	3 months	2 x 300 ml (10½ fl oz) jars

We covered mushroom preserving quite extensively in the first book, but this pickled mushroom recipe is so delicious we just had to include it here.

All mushrooms work well for pickling. We use Swiss brown, button or chestnut mushrooms, but you could also use pine mushrooms if you're lucky enough to find some. Just remember that pine mushrooms turn a bit gelatinous over time, so rinse them off before serving.

Pickled mushrooms are great in salads, pasta sauces and risotto, and as part of a shared plate. Try adding some, thinly sliced, to the mushroom salad on page 115.

PICKLED GARLICKY MUSHROOMS

250 ml (9 fl oz/1 cup) red
    wine vinegar
250 ml (9 fl oz/1 cup) water
55 g (2 oz/¼ cup) raw sugar
1 teaspoon salt
500 g (1 lb 2 oz) Swiss brown or
    button mushrooms
4 garlic cloves, peeled (see tip)
1 rosemary sprig, cut in half
2 thyme sprigs
½ teaspoon black peppercorns
vegetable oil or olive oil, for filling
    the jars (optional)

Make your brine by combining the vinegar, water, sugar and salt in a non-reactive, medium-sized saucepan. Place over low heat and stir to dissolve the sugar. Bring to simmering point, add the mushrooms and simmer in the brine for 2—5 minutes, or until softened slightly; be careful not to overcook.

Sterilise your jars and lids (see page 212).

When the jars are cool enough to handle, place 2 garlic cloves, ½ rosemary sprig, 1 thyme sprig and a few peppercorns into the bottom of each jar. Using a slotted spoon or tongs, remove the mushrooms from the brine and carefully but tightly pack them into the jars. Pour the hot brine over, making sure the mushrooms are completely submerged. If you like, you can top the mushrooms with a 1 cm (½ inch) layer of oil.

Remove any air bubbles by gently tapping each jar on the work surface and sliding a clean butter knife or chopstick around the inside to release any hidden air pockets. Wipe the rims of the jars with paper towel or a clean damp cloth and seal.

Store in the fridge for up to 3 months.

TIP: Garlic reacts to vinegar by turning blue. It's still edible, but can be a little unsettling to look at. If you wish to avoid this, blanch the garlic cloves for 10 seconds in boiling water before putting them in your jars.

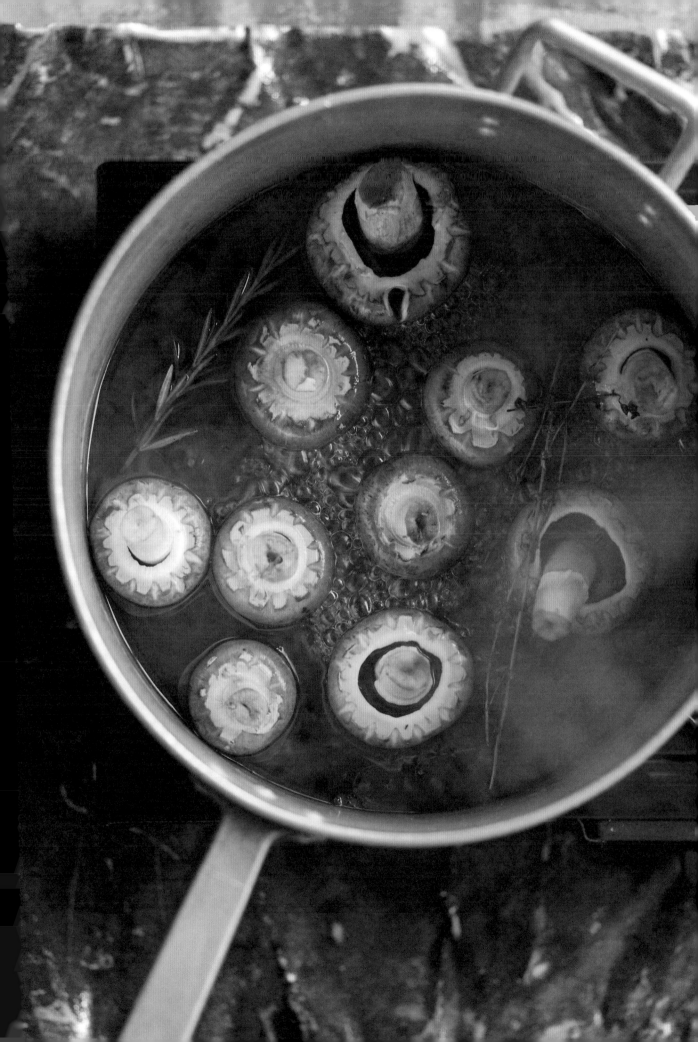

PREPARATION TIME	STORAGE	MAKES
20 minutes, plus 20 minutes sterilising, plus 10 minutes heat-processing	3 months, or up to 6 months if heat-processed	2 x 500 ml (17 fl oz/2 cup) jars

This recipe is a good one when you've got half a bunch of celery left over. We store these pickles in the fridge to keep them crisp and crunchy. Try thinly slicing them and tossing them through Tabouleh (see page 137) or grainy salads. Pickled celery is also amazing in a bloody mary!

PICKLED CELERY WITH LEMON & PEPPERCORNS

3–4 celery stalks (see tip)
250 ml (9 fl oz/1 cup) white wine vinegar
250 ml (9 fl oz/1 cup) water
55 g (2 oz/¼ cup) caster (superfine) sugar
½ teaspoon salt

FOR EACH JAR, YOU WILL NEED:
1 strip of lemon peel
1 bay leaf
3 black peppercorns
¼ teaspoon dill seeds
¼ teaspoon celery seeds

Wash the celery well and cut into strips or 5 cm (2 inch) chunks.

Sterilise your jars and lids (see page 212).

Make your brine by combining the vinegar, water, sugar and salt in a non-reactive, medium-sized saucepan. Place over low heat and stir to dissolve the sugar. Bring to the boil, then turn off the heat.

When the jars are cool enough to handle, add 1 lemon peel strip, 1 bay leaf and 3 peppercorns to the bottom of each jar. Add the dill and celery seeds, then carefully but tightly pack the raw celery in.

Cover with the hot brine, making sure the celery is completely submerged.

Remove any air bubbles by gently tapping each jar on the work surface and sliding a clean butter knife or chopstick around the inside to release any hidden air pockets. Wipe the rims of the jars with paper towel or a clean damp cloth and seal immediately.

We prefer to keep these pickles in the fridge as the cold helps them keep their crunch; they will keep in the fridge for 3 months.

To extend the shelf life to 6 months, heat-process the jars (see page 211) for 10 minutes, then store in a cool, dark place.

Once opened, refrigerate and use within 3 months.

TIP: Save the leaves from the celery stalks and use them in the Tabouleh recipe on page 137, or in the Vegie Scrap Bouillon on page 184.

PREPARATION TIME	STORAGE	MAKES
25 minutes, plus 20 minutes sterilising, plus 1–2 hours salting	3–6 months	3–4 x 200 ml (7 fl oz) jars

This tastes exactly like sushi-train ginger, only better! The ginger reacts to the vinegar and salt and turns a very pretty pink. Use this pickle thinly sliced through noodle salads, in dipping sauces or with sushi or fish.

GARI (JAPANESE-STYLE PICKLED GINGER)

There is no need to peel the ginger — just give it a good wash. Slice the ginger as finely as you can, using a mandoline or a very sharp knife. Place the ginger slices in a bowl and cover with the salt, mixing it through with your hands. Leave to stand for an hour or two.

Sterilise your jars and lids (see page 212).

Strain any excess water from the ginger slices and discard. Place the slices on a clean paper towel or tea towel and press out any excess salt and moisture.

Make your brine by combining the vinegar and sugar in a small non-reactive saucepan over low heat. Stir to dissolve the sugar and bring to simmering point.

When the jars are cool enough to handle, carefully pack the ginger into the warm jars.

Pour the hot brine over the ginger slices, making sure they are completely submerged.

Remove any air bubbles by gently tapping each jar on the work surface and sliding a clean butter knife or chopstick around the inside to release any hidden air pockets. Wipe the rims of the jars with paper towel or a clean damp cloth and seal immediately.

Leave to cool on the benchtop, then store in a cool, dark place for up to 3 months, or in the fridge for up to 6 months.

Once opened, refrigerate and use within 6 months.

400 g (14 oz) fresh ginger
2 tablespoons salt
500 ml (17 fl oz/2 cups) rice wine vinegar, with an acidity of at least 5%
110 g (3¾ oz/½ cup) caster (superfine) sugar

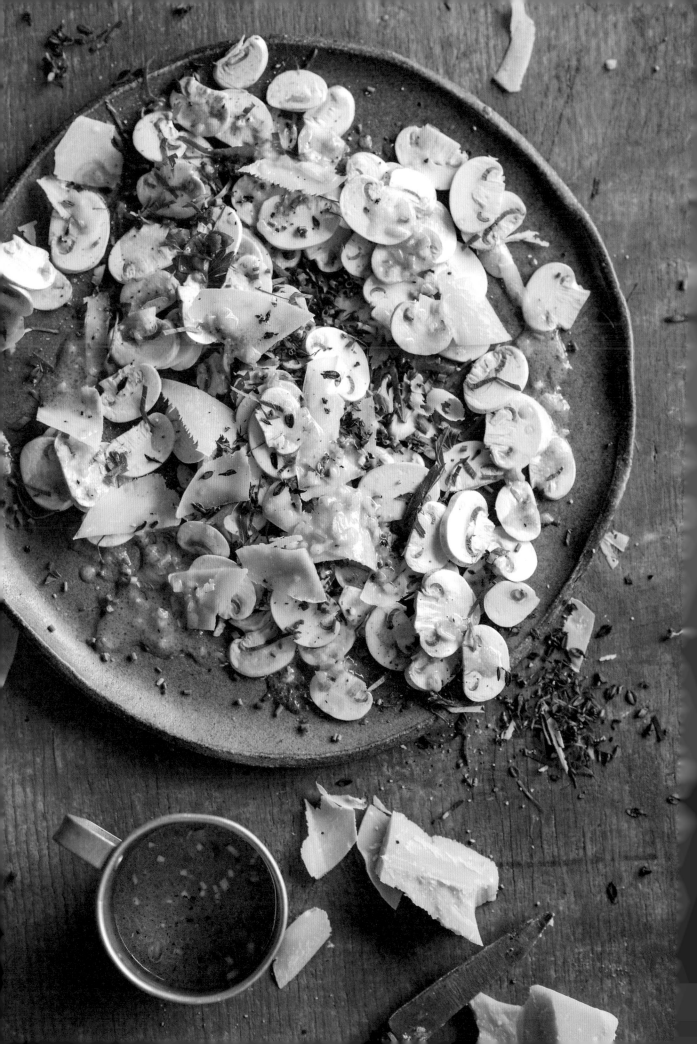

PREPARATION TIME	SERVES
20 minutes	4

To get the most from this simple salad, let the mushrooms sit in the dressing for 10–15 minutes before serving, to absorb the lovely flavours. It might seem like you have too much dressing, but you'll need it as mushrooms absorb so much liquid. Also try other herbs in this salad, such as tarragon and chervil.

RAW MUSHROOMS WITH CHIVES & MUSTARD

Using a very sharp knife, slice the mushrooms as thinly as you can. Place in a mixing bowl. Season with salt and pepper, add three-quarters of the herbs and let them sit while making the dressing.

Combine the vinegar, shallot and mustard in a small screw-top jar. Season with salt and pepper, add the olive oil, put the lid on and shake well to emulsify.

Place the mushrooms on a large serving plate. Pour the dressing on top and leave to sit for 10–15 minutes, if you have time; otherwise, you can serve immediately.

Just before serving, garnish with the remaining herbs and shaved parmesan.

400 g (14 oz) very fresh button mushrooms, or a mix of button and Swiss browns
1 tablespoon picked thyme leaves
1 small handful of picked flat-leaf (Italian) parsley leaves, thinly sliced
1 tablespoon finely snipped chives
60 ml (2 fl oz/¼ cup) sherry vinegar
1 French shallot, very finely chopped
2 teaspoons dijon mustard
80 ml (2½ fl oz/⅓ cup) olive oil
75 g (2½ oz) parmesan cheese, finely shaved

PREPARATION TIME	COOKING TIME	SERVES
20 minutes, plus 30 minutes salting	30 minutes, plus 15 minutes resting	4

We make our own miso at Cornersmith, and this dish is our version of the Japanese classic, miso eggplant. Sabine combines the eggplant with tofu and mustardy salad greens to make a delicious light autumn dish.

You could add brown rice, dressed with a little extra soy, sesame oil and lime juice, to turn it into a heartier meal.

GINGER & MISO-BRAISED EGGPLANT WITH TOFU, SPRING ONION & SESAME

1 large handful of mustard greens, or 2 handfuls of mizuna, washed and torn into pieces
125–150 g (4½–5½ oz) silken tofu, broken up a bit using a tablespoon
1 tablespoon sesame oil
juice of 1 lime
1½ teaspoons toasted sesame seeds (see page 206)
2 spring onions (scallions), thinly sliced
coriander (cilantro) leaves, to garnish (optional)

FOR THE EGGPLANT
1 largish eggplant (aubergine), about 500 g (1 lb 2 oz), cut into 2 cm (¾ inch) rounds
salt, for sprinkling
2 tablespoons miso paste
2 cm (¾ inch) knob of fresh ginger, peeled and finely grated
1 garlic clove, crushed
pinch of chilli powder
1 tablespoon rice wine vinegar
1 tablespoon sesame oil
1 tablespoon soy sauce
60 ml (2 fl oz/¼ cup) cooking-grade sake
30 g (1 oz) knob of butter, cut into small cubes

Start by preparing the eggplant. Sprinkle both sides of each eggplant slice with salt. Place them in a colander, set the colander on top of a bowl and leave to sit for about 30 minutes, to draw out the water and any bitterness.

Meanwhile, preheat the oven to 170°C (325°F).

Wash the salt off the eggplant and pat each slice dry with paper towel. Lay them in a baking dish large enough to fit them all in a single layer.

In a bowl, combine the miso paste, ginger, garlic, chilli powder, vinegar, sesame oil and soy sauce until smooth.

Spread the miso mixture evenly over the eggplant slices. Pour the sake and 60 ml (2 fl oz/¼ cup) water into the baking dish, to reach one-third to halfway up the side of the eggplant slices. Add the butter cubes.

Bake for about 30 minutes, or until the eggplant slices are cooked and soft, brushing them every 10 minutes with the braising liquid. Remove from the oven and leave to rest and cool in the braising liquid for a further 10–15 minutes.

Place the mustard leaves and tofu in a large mixing bowl and gently mix together. Season with salt and pepper and drizzle with the sesame oil and half the lime juice.

Place the dressed leaves on a large serving plate. Arrange the eggplant slices on top. Drizzle the braising liquid and remaining lime juice over the salad.

Garnish with the spring onion, sesame seeds and coriander, if using, and serve.

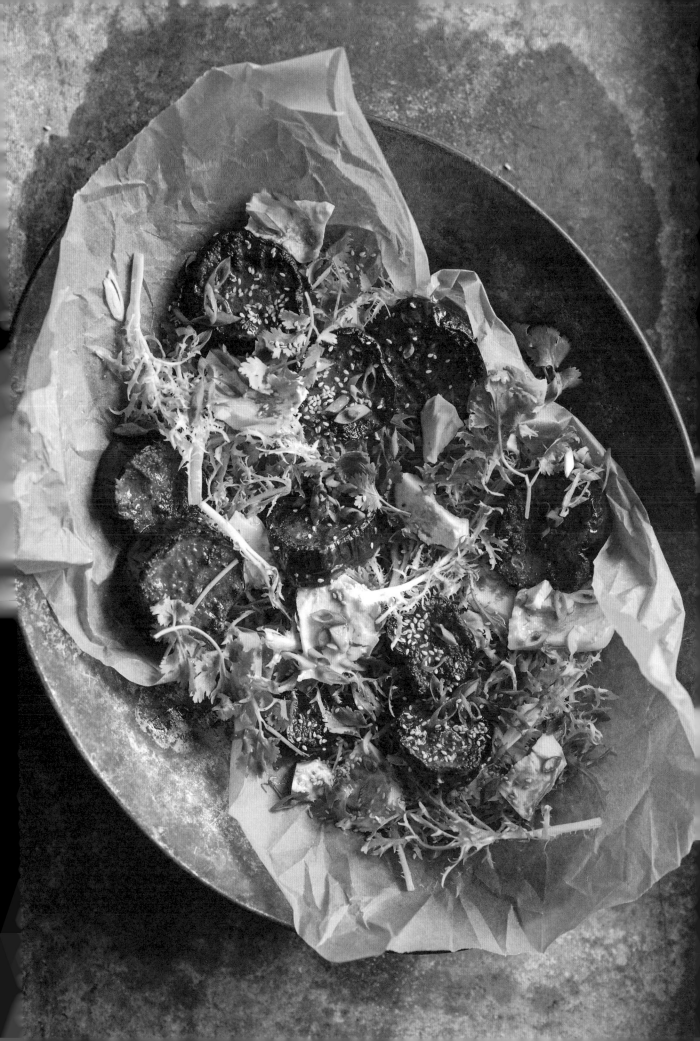

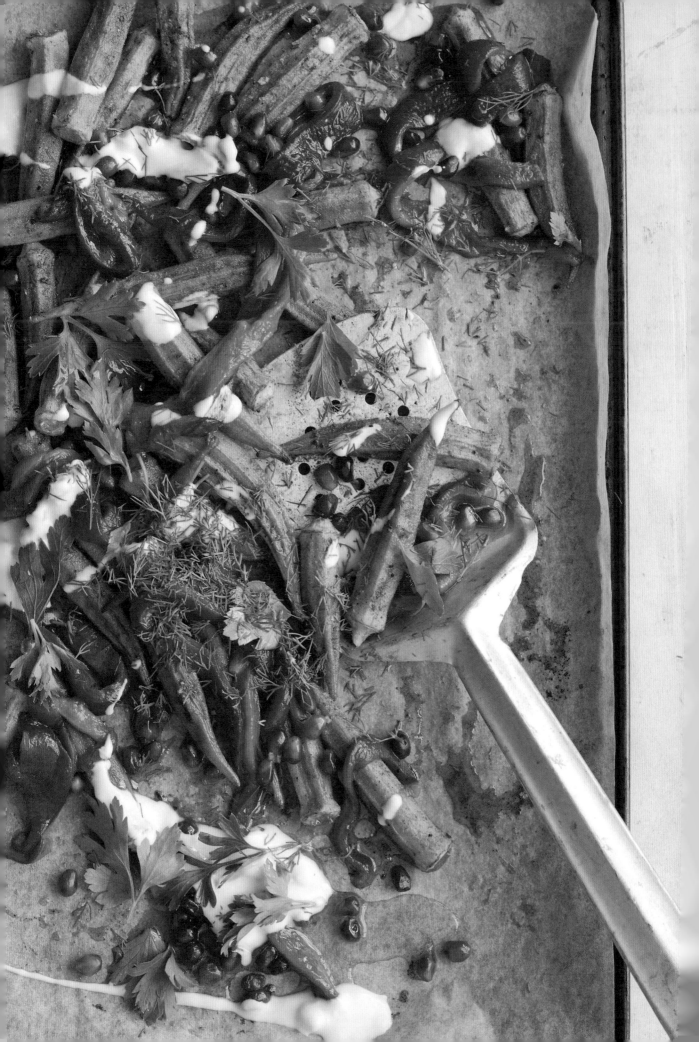

If you've never tried okra before, try this recipe — it's amazing. The roasted capsicum adds a bit of sweetness to this salad, balanced out by the acidity of yoghurt and the tartness of the pomegranate. Definitely give this one a go.

WHOLE ROASTED OKRA & CAPSICUM WITH POMEGRANATE, YOGHURT & HERBS

Preheat the oven to 200°C (400°F). Line a baking tray with baking paper.

Carefully wash and dry the okra, being careful not to break the skins. Place in a mixing bowl. Add the spices and salt, and enough olive oil to coat the okra, mixing gently.

Arrange the okra on the baking tray in one layer. Bake for 12 minutes.

Turn the oven onto its grill setting and grill the okra for another 2–3 minutes, to crisp up. Remove from the oven and leave to cool for a few minutes.

Combine the capsicum, pomegranate seeds and herbs in a large mixing bowl. Add the lemon juice and season with salt and pepper.

Add the roasted okra to the salad, then transfer to a large serving bowl or plate. Drizzle the yoghurt over the salad, finish with a drizzle of olive oil and serve.

400 g (14 oz) okra
¼ teaspoon sweet paprika
¼ teaspoon ground cumin
¼ teaspoon ground coriander
¼ teaspoon salt
2–3 tablespoons olive oil, plus extra for drizzling over the salad
150 g (5½ oz) roasted red capsicum (pepper), cut into thin strips (see tip)
1 pomegranate, broken into quarters, seeds separated
2 teaspoons finely chopped dill
1 handful of picked flat-leaf (Italian) parsley leaves
juice of 1 lemon
100 g (3½ oz) natural unsweetened yoghurt

TIP: You could roast some raw capsicum, if you have the time; for this recipe you will need 1 medium-sized raw capsicum, but you could roast several at the same time to use in other dishes. Set an oven rack near the top of your oven, beneath the element. Preheat the oven to 200°C (400°F). Place the whole capsicum/s on a baking tray and grill on the top oven rack for 10–15 minutes, turning every 3–4 minutes, until the skin is blistered all around. Place in a plastic bag and leave to cool in the fridge for 15–20 minutes. Peel off the skin, discard the seeds and white membranes, then use as desired. The roasted capsicum will keep, covered in oil, in an airtight jar in your fridge for up to 10 days, for you to use as needed.

PREPARATION TIME	STORAGE	MAKES
10 minutes, plus 20 minutes sterilising, plus 10 minutes heat-processing (optional)	3 months, or up to 1 year if heat-processed	2 x 500 ml (17 fl oz/2 cup) jars

This hot pickled okra is delicious, and adds a real punch of flavour and heat to any Mexican-style dishes. We often serve it with tortillas and beans, or thinly sliced through slaws.

Many people don't like the 'sliminess' of okra, which is due to its high mucilage content. If you keep the okra whole and are careful not to pierce or break the skin, the gooey mucilage will not leach out.

CHILLI-PICKLED OKRA

500 ml (17 fl oz/2 cups) white wine vinegar
250 ml (9 fl oz/1 cup) water
55 g (2 oz/¼ cup) sugar
1½ teaspoons salt
pinch of cayenne pepper
500 g (1 lb 2 oz) okra, washed

FOR EACH JAR, YOU WILL NEED:
1 garlic clove, peeled
2 slices fresh ginger
¼ teaspoon coriander seeds
¼ teaspoon black peppercorns
1 teaspoon chilli flakes, or 1 whole small chilli

Sterilise your jars and lids (see page 212).

Make your brine by combining the vinegar, water, sugar, salt and cayenne pepper in a non-reactive, medium-sized saucepan. Place over low heat and stir to dissolve the sugar and salt. Bring to simmering point, then turn off the heat.

When the jars are cool enough to handle, put the garlic, ginger, coriander seeds and peppercorns into the bottom of each jar.

Using small clean tongs or clean hands, carefully but tightly pack the raw whole okra in, packing them vertically, with some stems facing up and some stems facing down. Pour in the hot brine, making sure all the okra is completely submerged.

Remove any air bubbles by gently tapping each jar on the work surface and sliding a clean butter knife or chopstick around the inside to release any hidden air pockets. Wipe the rims of the jars with paper towel or a clean damp cloth and seal immediately.

Leave to cool on the benchtop, then store in the fridge for up to 3 months, or heat-process for 10 minutes and store in a cool, dark place for up to 1 year.

Allow to sit for at least 2 weeks before eating. Once opened, refrigerate and use within 6 months.

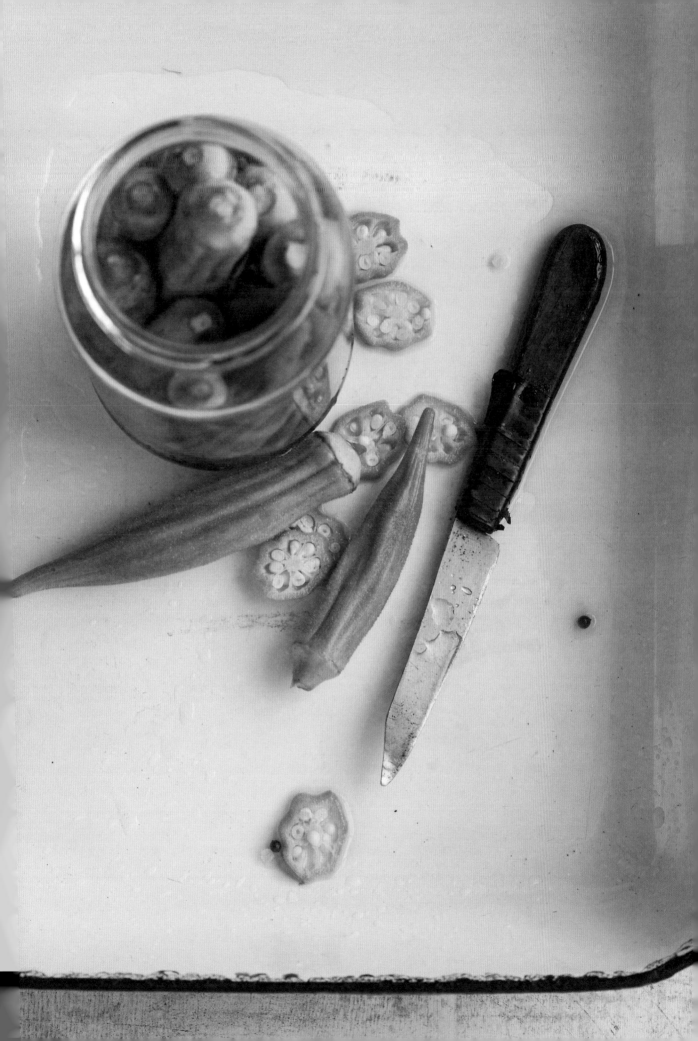

PREPARATION TIME	COOKING TIME	SERVES
20 minutes, plus at least 8 hours soaking	1 hour, plus 20 minutes resting	4

There are so many delicious bean varieties available in autumn; here we use green beans and snake beans, but you could also use yellow wax beans or flat roman beans. In this salad we combine them with garlic, lemon and mint — a classic combination of Italian flavours.

This is quite a light bean salad, with the added crunch of bean sprouts. You can use any bean or lentil-based sprout here — or better still, sprout your own! It's really easy and fun to do at home with kids. See pages 130–131.

THREE-BEAN SALAD WITH SPROUTS, MINT & GARLIC DRESSING

200–250 g (7–9 oz) green beans
200–250 g (7–9 oz) snake (long) beans
100 g (3½ oz) bean sprouts, such as adzuki or chickpea
1 teaspoon finely chopped preserved lemon or lime rind (or Salt-preserved citrus skins on page 187)
1 teaspoon picked thyme leaves
1 handful of picked mint leaves
1 tablespoon picked dill leaves

FOR THE WHITE BEANS
100 g (3½ oz) dried white beans, soaked for 8 hours, or overnight
1 garlic clove, peeled
1 bay leaf
1 thyme sprig
2–3 black peppercorns
1 teaspoon sea salt

GARLIC DRESSING
1½ tablespoons white wine vinegar
½ teaspoon dijon mustard
½ teaspoon wholegrain mustard
1 garlic clove, crushed
60 ml (2 fl oz/¼ cup) olive oil

Start by cooking the white beans. Drain and rinse them, then place in a large saucepan and add enough fresh water to cover them by 5 cm (2 inches). Add the garlic, bay leaf, thyme sprig and peppercorns and bring slowly to the boil. Skim off any foam, reduce the heat and leave to gently simmer for 45–60 minutes, or until the beans are tender but still retain their shape, gently stirring them occasionally.

When the beans are cooked, take them off the heat, add the salt, put the lid on and let them sit for 15–20 minutes to absorb the salt.

Meanwhile, bring a large saucepan of salted water to the boil. Top and tail the green beans and snake beans, then blanch both bean varieties separately for about 2 minutes, or until just cooked but still crunchy. Refresh in iced water, drain well, then cut them diagonally in half.

Place the fresh beans in a large mixing bowl. Add the sprouts, preserved lemon and most of the thyme, dill and mint. Mix well.

To make the dressing, combine the vinegar, mustards and garlic in a small screw-top jar. Season with salt and pepper. Mix well, then add the olive oil, put the lid on and shake well until emulsified.

Drain the white beans, reserving the liquid (see tip) and add them to the salad. Add the dressing and mix gently.

Arrange the salad in a serving bowl, garnish with the remaining herbs and serve.

TIP: Keep your bean cooking liquid to make a bean soup in autumn or winter. Just freeze it and use it as a stock the next time you are making a bean or lentil-based soup.

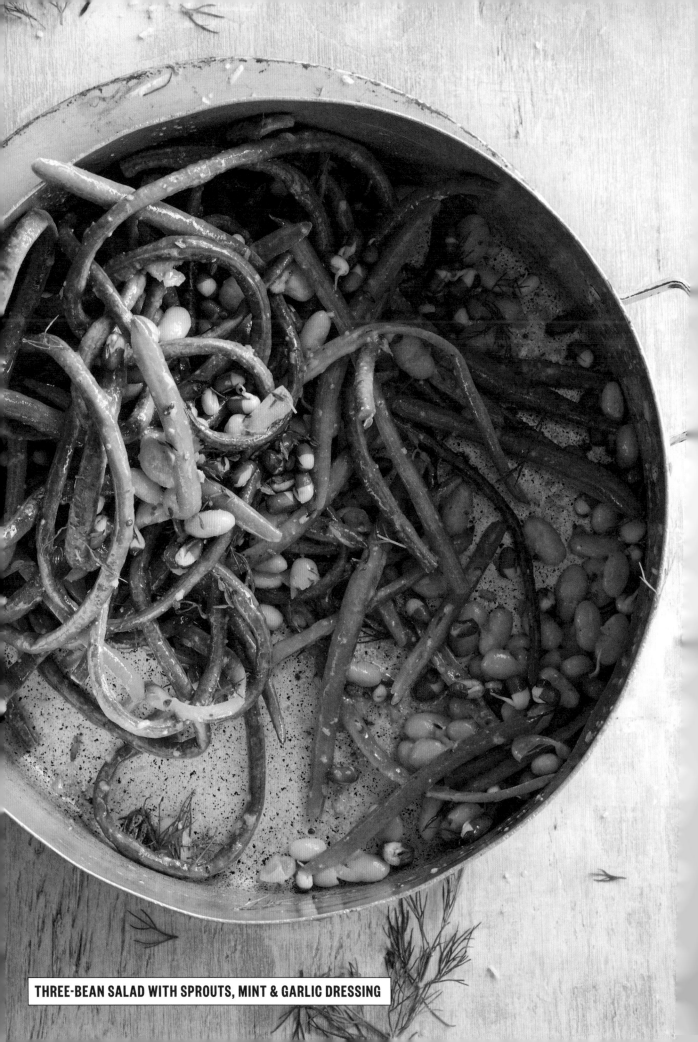

THREE-BEAN SALAD WITH SPROUTS, MINT & GARLIC DRESSING

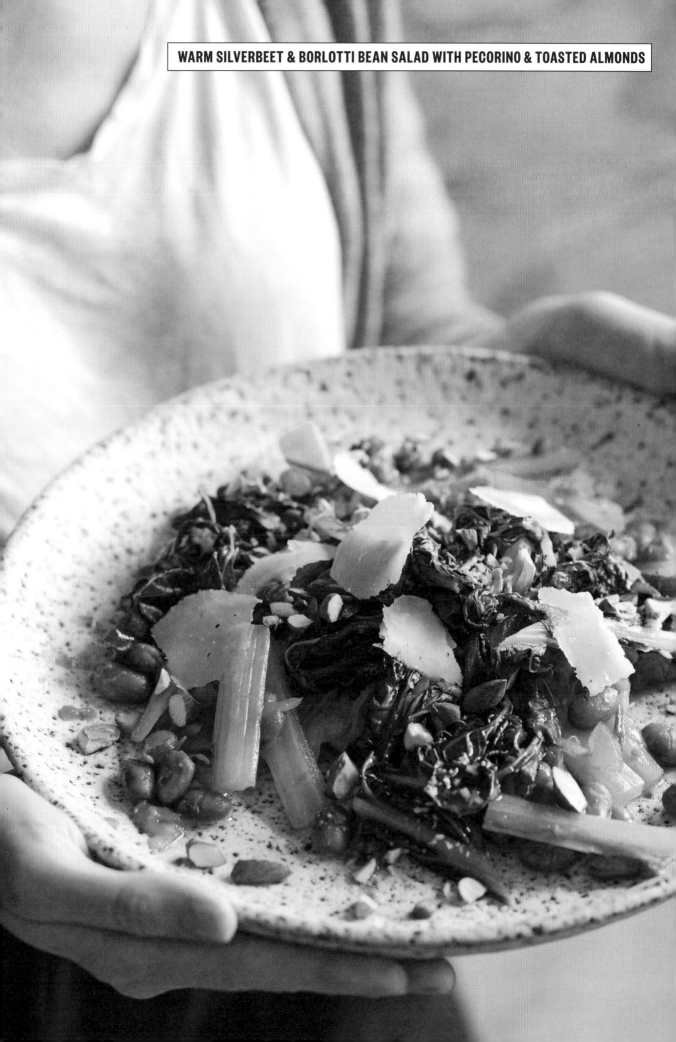

PREPARATION TIME	COOKING TIME	SERVES
25 minutes, plus at least 8 hours soaking	1¼ hours, plus 20 minutes resting	4

This is a very hearty, warming salad for the cooler months. A soft-boiled egg would make a wonderful accompaniment, and turn it into a complete meal.

You can lighten it up a little by keeping the silverbeet raw and massaging salt into the raw silverbeet leaves (as you do with the kale in the nashi pear and kale salad on page 106), and leaving out the garlic.

If you can get your hands on fresh borlotti beans, it will greatly reduce your cooking time (to around 20–25 minutes), and you won't need to soak them either.

WARM SILVERBEET & BORLOTTI BEAN SALAD WITH PECORINO & TOASTED ALMONDS

generous pinch of saffron threads
1 small bunch silverbeet (Swiss chard), about 450 g (1 lb)
2½ tablespoons olive oil, plus extra for drizzling over the salad
1 brown onion, thinly sliced
3 garlic cloves, crushed, plus 1 sliced garlic clove
2 very ripe tomatoes, finely chopped
1 large red chilli, seeded and thinly sliced
1 tablespoon olive oil
zest and juice of 1–2 lemons
40 g (1½ oz/¼ cup) toasted almonds (see page 206), chopped
40 g (1½ oz/½ cup) shaved pecorino (see tip)

FOR THE BEANS
100 g (3½ oz) dried borlotti beans (see tip), soaked for 8 hours, or overnight
1 garlic clove, smashed with the back of a knife
1 brown onion, peeled and cut in half
1 thyme sprig
1 teaspoon sea salt

Start by cooking the borlotti beans. Drain and rinse them, then place in a large saucepan and add enough fresh water to cover them by 5 cm (2 inches). Add the garlic, onion halves and thyme sprig and bring slowly to the boil. Skim off any foam, reduce the heat and leave to gently simmer for 45–60 minutes, or until the beans are tender but still retain their shape, gently stirring them occasionally.

When the beans are cooked, take them off the heat, add the salt, put the lid on and let them sit for about 15–20 minutes to absorb the salt.

Meanwhile, put the saffron in a small heatproof bowl, add 125 ml (4 fl oz/½ cup) boiling water and leave to steep for 10 minutes.

Prepare the silverbeet by cutting the leaves from the stems. Set the leaves aside. Trim the silverbeet stems, peel off any fibrous bits, and cut the stems into chunky batons.

Heat the olive oil in a heavy-based saucepan over medium heat. Add the onion and crushed garlic. Season with salt and cook the onion for about 5 minutes, until aromatic and soft. Add the silverbeet stems, tomato and chilli and cook for another 2–3 minutes, then stir in the 'saffron water'. Cover and simmer for 15 minutes.

Drain the borlotti beans and stir them through the tomato mixture. Cook for a further 5–7 minutes, or until the silverbeet stems are soft and juicy.

Meanwhile, cut the reserved silverbeet leaves into large bite-sized pieces. Heat a large frying pan over medium–high heat. Add the olive oil, then the silverbeet leaves. Season with salt and pepper and stir for a few minutes, until they start wilting.

Add the lemon zest and sliced garlic, and stir for 2–3 minutes, until the garlic has softened. Transfer the mixture to a bowl, add the lemon juice and season to taste.

Place the braised borlotti bean mixture on a serving plate, then arrange the silverbeet leaf mixture on top. Scatter the almonds and shaved pecorino over and finish with an extra drizzle of olive oil.

TIP: If you happen to have a piece of pecorino (or parmesan) with the rind on, you can put the rind into the bean cooking liquid, or put it under olive oil and let it sit for a while. The oil will take on the 'cheesy' flavour beautifully, and can be used in cooking, salads or for finishing dishes.

PREPARATION TIME	COOKING TIME	STORAGE	MAKES
25 minutes, plus at least 2 hours salting, plus 20 minutes sterilising, plus 15 minutes heat-processing (optional)	45 minutes	1 month, or up to 1 year if heat-processed	2 x 500 ml (17 fl oz/2 cup) jars

This is more of an antipasto-style pickle. It's so delicious you'll probably just eat it straight out of the jar, but it is lovely with soft cheeses or as part of a tasting plate for lunch. You could also serve it as a side with grilled fish, or tossed through leafy salads.

PICKLED ROASTED FENNEL

2 small fennel bulbs, about 500 g (1 lb 2 oz) in total
1 onion
80 ml (2½ fl oz/⅓ cup) vegetable oil or olive oil
1 teaspoon fennel seeds
1 teaspoon salt
300 ml (10½ fl oz) white wine vinegar
150 ml (5 fl oz) water
110 g (3¾ oz/½ cup) caster (superfine) sugar
2 garlic cloves, peeled
½ teaspoon black peppercorns
2 bay leaves

Preheat the oven to 180°C (350°F). Slice the fennel into long wedges and thinly slice the onion. Put the vegetables in a baking dish. Drizzle with the oil, sprinkle with the fennel seeds and salt and mix together.

Roast for 30–45 minutes, or until the fennel is soft, sweet and starting to brown on the edges.

Meanwhile, sterilise your jars and lids (see page 212).

Make your brine by combining the vinegar, water and sugar in a non-reactive, medium-sized saucepan. Place over low heat and stir to dissolve the sugar. Increase the heat and bring to the boil.

When the jars are cool enough to handle, put 1 garlic clove, a few peppercorns and 1 bay leaf into the bottom of each jar. Use a pair of small clean tongs or clean hands to carefully pack the roasted fennel and onion into the jars. Cover with the hot brine, making sure the vegetables are completely submerged.

Remove any air bubbles by gently tapping each jar on the work surface and sliding a clean butter knife or chopstick around the inside to release any hidden air pockets. Wipe the rims of the jars with paper towel or a clean damp cloth and seal immediately.

Leave to cool on the benchtop, then store in the fridge for up to 1 month. To extend the shelf life to 1 year, heat-process the jars (see page 211) for 15 minutes.

Once opened, refrigerate and use within 3 months.

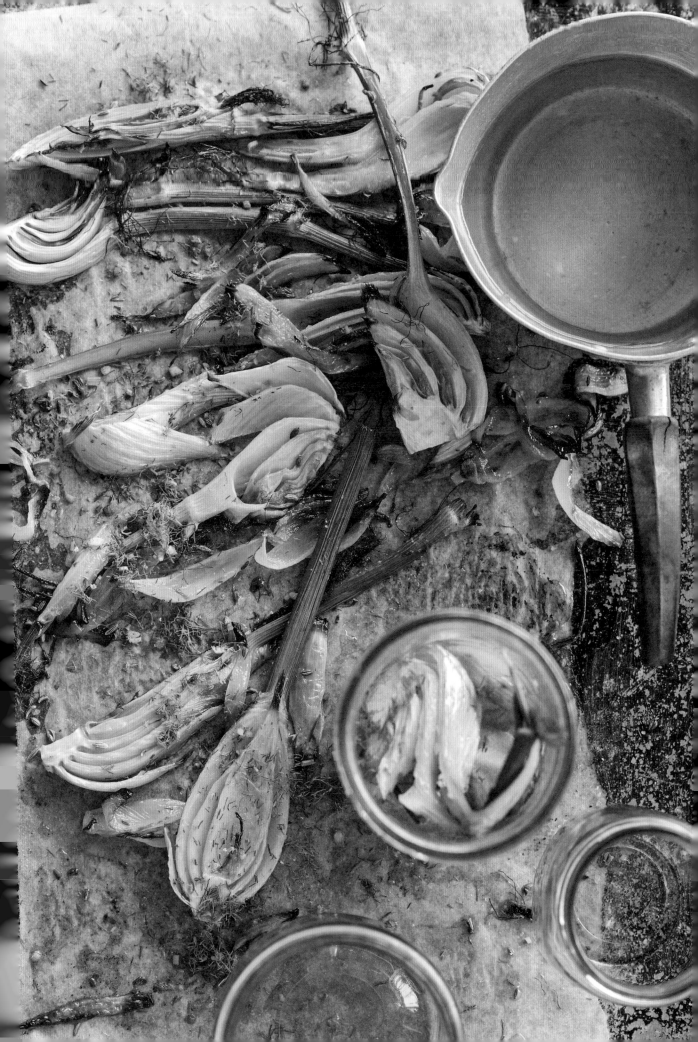

SPROUTING

Sprouted pulses, seeds and grains are little power packs of nutrition. They're a great source of vitamins and provide their own enzymes, making them easy for the body to digest. As a protein source, sprouted pulses are a valuable addition to vegetarian dishes.

Sprouts also add texture, colour and flavour to salads and sandwiches, as well as soups and other warm dishes — just be sure to only heat them very gently, to preserve their goodness.

Growing your own sprouts provides a fresh, clean, living food, available throughout the seasons, and is very easy to do.

The simple method outlined here requires no special equipment, and is suitable for chickpeas, whole lentils, mung beans, black-eyed peas, green peas and grains. As sprouting times are similar, a combination of pulses can be sprouted in one container. The yield of sprouts will be double the volume of dry ingredient.

We recommend using organic local pulses for sprouting.

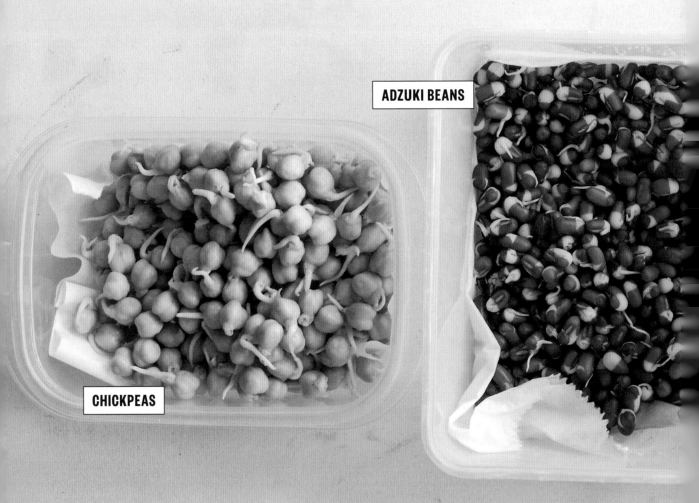

ADZUKI BEANS

CHICKPEAS

Sprouting at home is quite straightforward, but you do need to be careful not to expose the sprouts to fluctuating temperatures, as this will affect their ability to germinate.

Sprouts grow best at a relatively stable ambient room temperature, so if you live in an area that has very hot summers, you should restrict your sprouting season to autumn, winter and early spring.

Similarly, if your winters are very cold your seeds may struggle to germinate and grow unless you can keep them in a relatively warm, temperature-controlled spot.

To start with, place your chosen grains or pulses in a deep bowl and cover with cold water – 2 parts water to 1 part dry ingredient. Leave your grains to soak and absorb the water for 2–4 hours, and pulses for 8–10 hours.

Using a sieve or colander, drain the excess water from the soaked grains or pulses, then rinse them thoroughly under a cold tap until the water runs clear.

Drain again, taking time to allow as much water as possible to drain off. It is important that your sprouts and grains don't sit in any water, as undesirable micro-organisms may start breeding in the water, and your sprouts may become mouldy.

Place the sieve or colander over a deep bowl. Cover it with a light cloth or tea towel, to protect from dust and insects. Leave on the kitchen benchtop, at room temperature, away from direct sunlight, for 8–10 hours.

Over the next 2–3 days, rinse and drain your sprouts twice daily. Your sprouts are ready to eat as soon as the shoots are visible, but you can grow them as short or as long as you like.

When you're happy with their length, store them in the fridge in a sealed container and you'll have fresh sprouts for the week.

Take out portions as you need them, and avoid leaving them out on the bench.

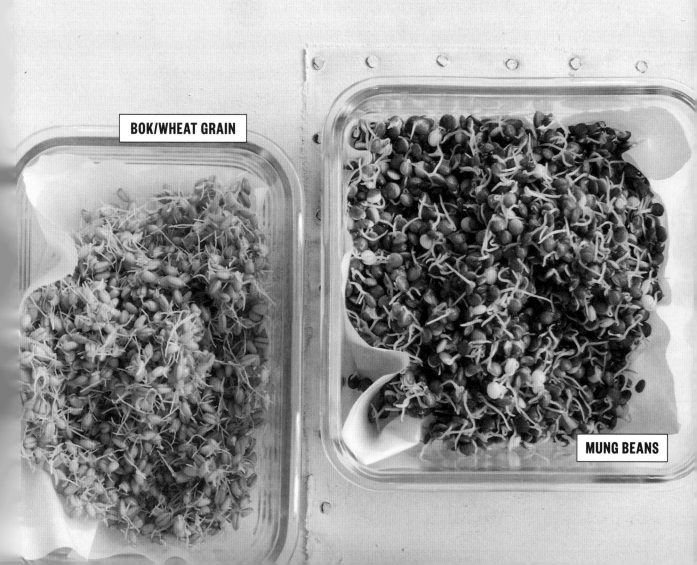

BOK/WHEAT GRAIN

MUNG BEANS

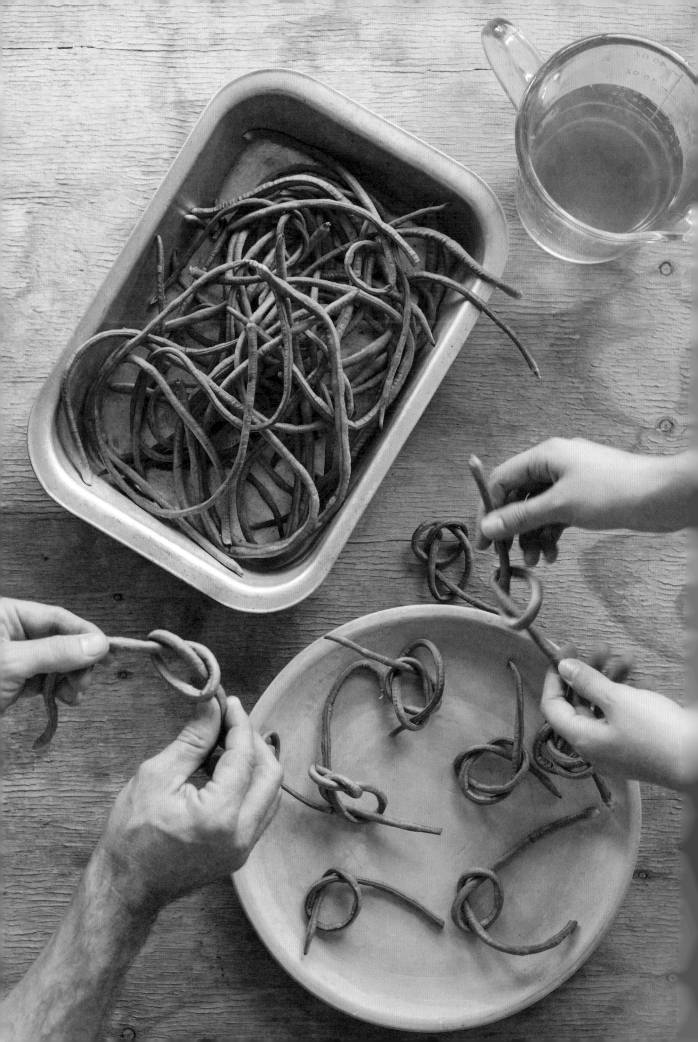

PREPARATION TIME	STORAGE	MAKES
20 minutes, plus 20 minutes sterilising	3 months	1 x 750 ml (26 fl oz) jar

Green beans make great pickles! And these knotted snake bean pickles are delicious and adorable. They are best kept in the fridge, as snake beans tend to get a bit slimy over time.

KNOTTED SNAKE BEAN PICKLES

Sterilise your jar and lid (see page 212).

Wash the beans and trim off any blemished ends. Tie any long beans into loose knots or coils.

Make your brine by combining the vinegar, water, sugar, salt and turmeric in a non-reactive, medium-sized saucepan. Place over low heat and stir to dissolve the sugar and salt. Bring to simmering point, add your knotted beans and blanch for 2–3 minutes, then turn off the heat.

When the jar is cool enough to handle, put the peppercorns and dill seeds in the bottom. Add the garlic and chilli flakes, if using, then carefully pack the beans in. Add the hot brine (see tip), making sure the beans are completely submerged.

Remove any air bubbles by gently tapping the jar on the work surface and sliding a clean butter knife or chopstick around the inside to release any hidden air pockets. Wipe the rim of the jar with paper towel or a clean damp cloth and seal immediately.

They will keep in the fridge for up to 3 months.

___

TIP: Any leftover brine can be stored in the fridge for up to 1 month and used for pickling and quick-pickling, or as a base for salad dressings.

1 big bunch snake (long) beans, about 300–400 g (10½–14 oz)
500 ml (17 fl oz/2 cups) white wine vinegar
250 ml (9 fl oz/1 cup) water
75 g (2½ oz/⅓ cup) sugar
1 teaspoon salt
¼ teaspoon ground turmeric
½ teaspoon black peppercorns
1 teaspoon dill seeds
2 garlic cloves, peeled
1 teaspoon chilli flakes (optional)

PREPARATION TIME	COOKING TIME	STORAGE	MAKES
40 minutes, plus 20 minutes sterilising, plus 10 minutes heat-processing (optional)	about 1 hour	6 months, or up to 2 years if heat-processed	3–4 x 300 ml (10½ fl oz) jars

Limes are one of our favourite fruits, and lime pickle is one of our favourite autumn preserves. As soon as lime season takes off and the price drops, we start bottling! This pickle is wonderful with curries, seafood and fried eggs. You can also mix a tablespoon through yoghurt to make a flavoursome marinade for chicken or fish.

LIME PICKLE

1 kg (2 lb 4 oz) limes (preferably unwaxed)
80 ml (2½ fl oz/⅓ cup) vegetable oil
500 g (1 lb 2 oz) onions, thinly sliced
3–4 garlic cloves, crushed
375 ml (13 fl oz/1½ cups) white wine vinegar
110 g (3¾ oz/½ cup) sugar
1 tablespoon salt
1 teaspoon fenugreek seeds, toasted and ground (see tip)
2 teaspoons cumin seeds, toasted and ground (see tip)
2 teaspoons coriander seeds, toasted and ground (see tip)
1–2 teaspoons chilli flakes
½ teaspoon ground turmeric
6–8 curry leaves

Put the limes in a saucepan with 3 litres (105 fl oz/ 12 cups) water. Simmer over medium heat for 20–30 minutes, or until soft.

Strain the limes, then leave to cool slightly. Cut the limes into very thin strips, or finely dice them. Set aside in a bowl, making sure you add all the lime pulp.

Heat the vegetable oil in a large non-reactive saucepan. Sauté the onion over medium heat for about 8 minutes, until soft, translucent and sweet. Add the garlic and sauté for another minute or two, until fragrant.

Turn the heat down to low. Add the lime mixture, vinegar, sugar, salt, spices and curry leaves, stirring to combine. Simmer for 15 minutes, or until the sauce thickens, stirring often so it doesn't stick to the pan. Don't let it dry out too much, as you need moisture to cover the limes once they're packed into the jars.

Meanwhile, sterilise your jars and lids (see page 212).

Carefully fill the hot jars with the hot pickle. Remove any air bubbles by sliding a clean butter knife around the inside to release any hidden air pockets. Wipe the rims of the jars with paper towel and seal immediately.

Leave to cool on the benchtop, then store in a cool, dark place for up to 6 months. To extend the shelf life to 2 years, heat-process the jars (see page 211) for 10 minutes. Let the lime pickle sit for at least 2 months before eating; it will be even better after 6 months.

Once opened, refrigerate and use within 6 months.

TIP: To toast the spice seeds, gently fry them in a small frying pan without any oil for a minute or two, until aromatic, stirring constantly so they don't burn. It's best to toast them separately, as fenugreek seeds need only a very quick fry to avoid bitterness. Grind to a powder using a spice grinder or mortar and pestle.

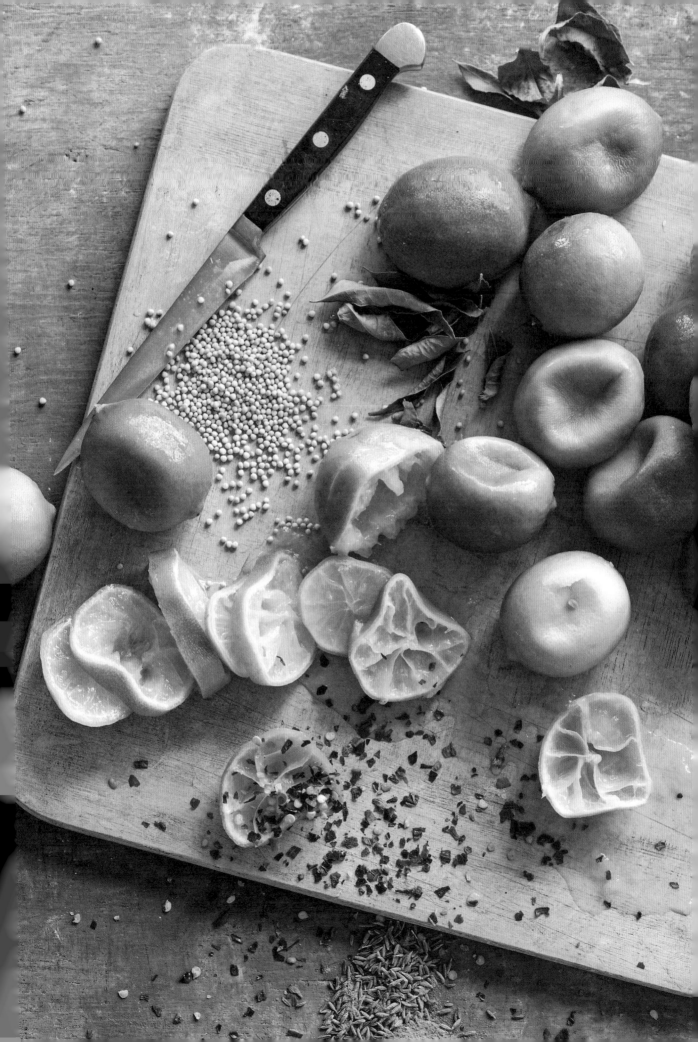

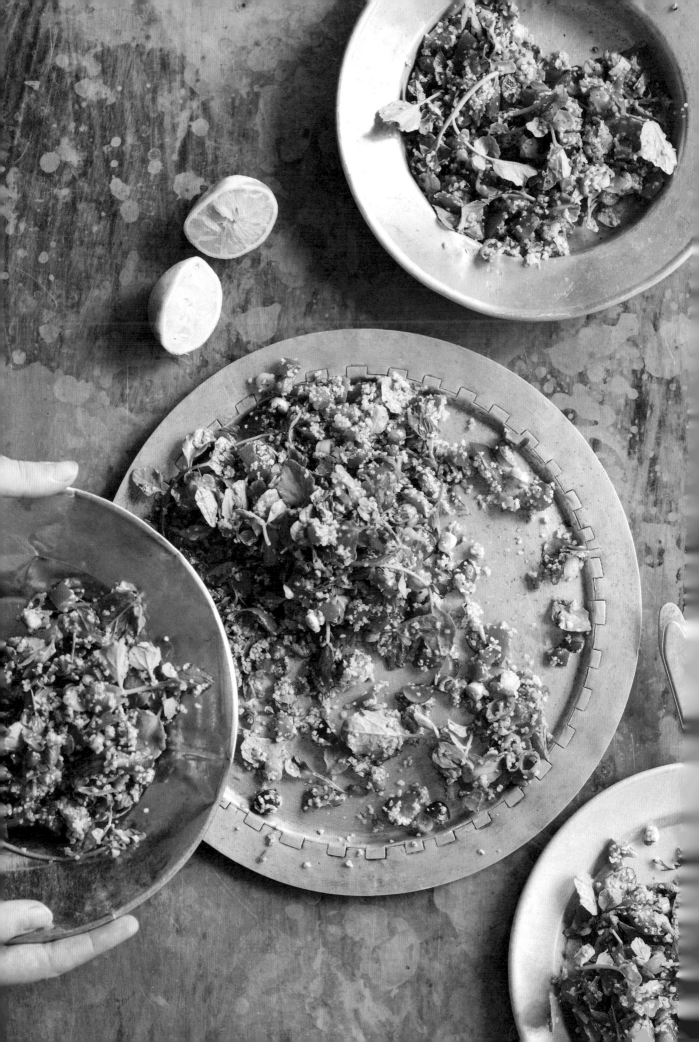

PREPARATION TIME	SERVES
20 minutes, plus 15 minutes soaking	4

This simple tabouleh is basically a 'no waste' salad, using up whatever vegetables you have in your fridge, combining them with lots of fragrant herbs such as parsley, mint or dill, a small amount of cracked wheat, some spices, and lots of lemon or lime juice and olive oil. Experiment with ingredients such as watercress, endive, radicchio, grapes, pomegranate, Pickled Celery (page 112), Pickled Green Tomatoes (page 20), pickled cucumber, chilli …

The vegetables and herbs can easily be prepared ahead of time. Just be sure to dress the salad just before serving.

TABOULEH WITH WATERCRESS & GRAPES

Rinse the burghul and place in a bowl. Add 250 ml (9 fl oz/ 1 cup) water and leave to soak for 15 minutes.

Place the watercress, herbs, tomatoes, grapes, spring onion and citrus zest in a large serving bowl.

Drain any excess water from the burghul. Place the burghul in a clean tea towel and twist the ends to squeeze the burghul dry.

Add the burghul to the salad bowl. Add the spices, citrus juice and olive oil. Season with salt and pepper, mix well and serve.

100 g (3½ oz/½ cup) burghul (bulgur)
1 large handful of picked watercress sprigs
1 handful of picked mint leaves, finely shredded
1 handful of picked flat-leaf (Italian) parsley leaves, finely shredded
4 ripe tomatoes, (or 2 red and 2 Pickled Green Tomatoes from page 20), cut into very small dice
90 g (3¼ oz/½ cup) grapes, cut into very small dice
2 spring onions (scallions), thinly sliced
zest of 1 lemon or lime
¼ teaspoon ground allspice
¼ teaspoon ground cinnamon
pinch of chilli flakes or powder
juice of 2 lemons or limes
100 ml (3½ fl oz) olive oil, approximately

PREPARATION TIME	COOKING TIME	STORAGE	MAKES
45 minutes, plus 20 minutes sterilising, plus 10 minutes heat-processing	1¼ hours	Up to 2 years	4 x 300 ml (10½ fl oz) jars

This chutney is a good one to make at the end of plum season, when there's an abundance of cheap, delicious plums around. We also use this recipe for summer stone fruits — peaches, nectarines and apricots all make yummy chutneys. You can use apple cider vinegar or red wine vinegar if you prefer; just remember your vinegars need to be 5% acidity or more for preserving.

PLUM & GINGER CHUTNEY

1.5 kg (3 lb 5 oz) plums
500 g (1 lb 2 oz) onions
80 ml (2½ fl oz/⅓ cup) vegetable oil
60 g (2¼ oz/⅓ cup) grated fresh ginger
1 teaspoon brown or yellow mustard seeds
½ teaspoon chilli flakes
¼ teaspoon ground cloves, or 3 whole cloves
½ teaspoon ground cinnamon
250 ml (9 fl oz/1 cup) white wine vinegar
110 g (3¾ oz/½ cup) raw sugar
1 teaspoon salt
½ teaspoon freshly ground black pepper

Cut the plums into 2 cm (¾ inch) cubes and discard the stones. Thinly slice the onions.

Heat the vegetable oil in a large non-reactive saucepan and sauté the onion over medium heat for about 8 minutes, until soft and collapsed. Add the ginger and spices and stir for another minute or two, until fragrant. Add the plums and stir until the onion, plums and spices are evenly mixed. Add the vinegar, sugar and salt, stirring until the sugar and salt have dissolved.

Reduce the heat to low, stirring regularly to make sure the chutney isn't sticking. Cook for about 1 hour, until the desired consistency is reached. The chutney should be glossy and thick, with no puddles of liquid on top. Taste halfway through and add more spices or salt if needed; if your plums are very tart, you can add an extra 3 tablespoons or so of raw or brown sugar.

Meanwhile, sterilise your jars and lids (see page 212), putting the jars in the oven about 15 minutes before the chutney has finished cooking.

Carefully ladle the hot chutney into the hot jars.

Remove any air bubbles by gently tapping each jar on the work surface and sliding a clean butter knife or chopstick around the inside to release any hidden air pockets. Wipe the rims of the jars with paper towel or a clean damp cloth and seal immediately.

Heat-process the jars (see page 211) for 10 minutes, then store in a cool, dark place for up to 2 years.

Leave to sit for 2–3 months before eating; this chutney gets better and better with time.

Once opened, refrigerate and use within 6 months.

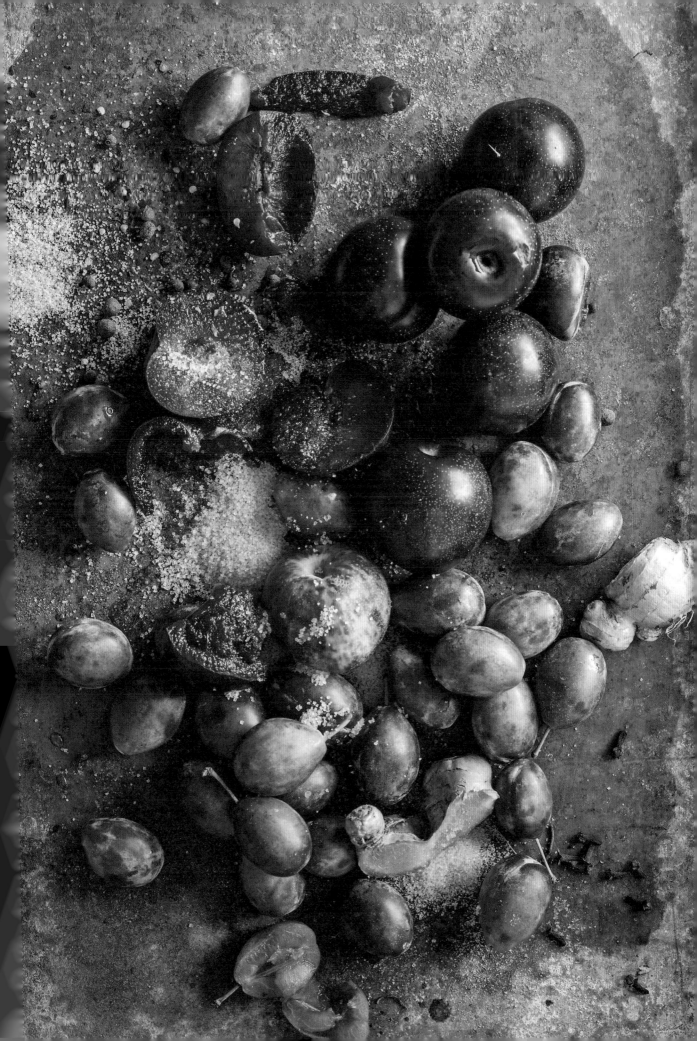

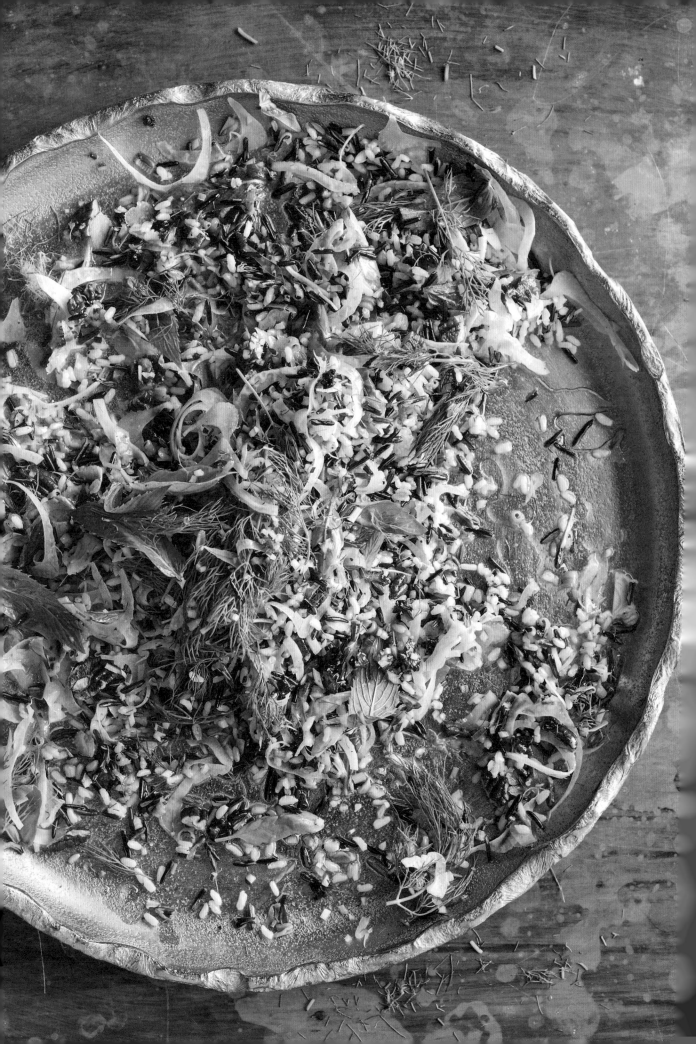

PREPARATION TIME	COOKING TIME	SERVES
20 minutes, plus at least 6 hours soaking	30 minutes	4

This salad draws inspiration from the pilaf rice dishes from Turkey and the Middle East. Soaking the brown rice before cooking it helps retain some of its bite, shape and texture, and stops the grains bursting and turning too mushy. We recommend cooking any grains you are using in salads this way.

If you haven't made the Stone Fruit Kernel Vinegar from page 166 yet, use sherry or red wine vinegar in the dressing. But be sure to try out the vinegar infused with prune kernels — it is delicious, and extracts a beautiful flavour from an item that would normally be thrown out.

WILD & BROWN RICE SALAD WITH FENNEL, PECANS, PRUNES & HERBS

Wash and drain the brown rice. Bring a large saucepan of salted water to the boil. Add the brown rice and gently boil for 8–12 minutes, or until the rice is just cooked, but still has a bite. Strain the rice, reserving the cooking water, and set aside to cool.

Pour the reserved cooking water into a large clean saucepan and bring it back to the boil. Add the wild rice and let it gently simmer for 10–12 minutes, or until just cooked. Wash and drain the wild rice, then leave to cool.

Combine the onion, fennel and prunes in a large mixing bowl. When the brown and wild rice have cooled, add them to the bowl and season generously with salt and pepper.

To make the dressing, combine the vinegar and honey in a small screw-top jar. Season with salt and pepper, add the olive oil, put the lid on and shake well to combine.

Add the herbs and pecans to the salad, pour the dressing over and gently combine until all the ingredients are coated with the dressing.

Arrange the salad in a serving bowl, sprinkle with the star anise and serve immediately.

200–220 g (7–8 oz/1 cup) short or medium-grain brown rice, soaked in water for 6–8 hours
200 g (7 oz/1 cup) wild rice, soaked in water for 6–8 hours
1 small red onion, finely diced
½ fennel bulb (or 1 small one), finely diced, or thinly sliced using a mandoline
4 prunes, pitted and finely diced
1½–2 tablespoons Stone Fruit Kernel Vinegar (see page 166), made using prune pits
1 teaspoon honey
3–4 tablespoons olive oil
1 large handful of mixed picked herbs, such as basil, dill and mint
50 g (1¾ oz/½ cup) toasted pecans (see page 206)
pinch of ground star anise

PREPARATION TIME	STORAGE	MAKES
20 minutes	uo to 1 month	1 x 1 litre (35 fl oz) container

Here's the perfect pickle when you've bought a whole cabbage for a slaw and end up having some left over in the bottom of your fridge. It's super easy to prepare, full of flavour, and makes mid-week sausages and mash a lot more appealing. Serve it sliced with pulled pork, or thinly sliced and tossed through salads for extra tang.

QUICK PICKLED CABBAGE WEDGES

½ small red cabbage,
    cut into wedges
500 ml (17 fl oz/2 cups)
    red wine vinegar
375 ml (13 fl oz/1½ cups) water
110 g (3¾ oz/½ cup) sugar
1 teaspoon caraway seeds
1 teaspoon black peppercorns
½ teaspoon juniper berries

Slice the cabbage into large 5 cm (2 inch) wedges.

Make your brine by combining the vinegar, water and sugar in a non-reactive, medium-sized saucepan. Place over low heat and stir to dissolve the sugar. Add the spices and bring to the boil.

Put your cabbage wedges in a heatproof glass container and cover with the hot brine.

Allow to cool, then seal and store in the fridge for up to 1 month. It will take about 3–4 days for the wedges to be pickled.

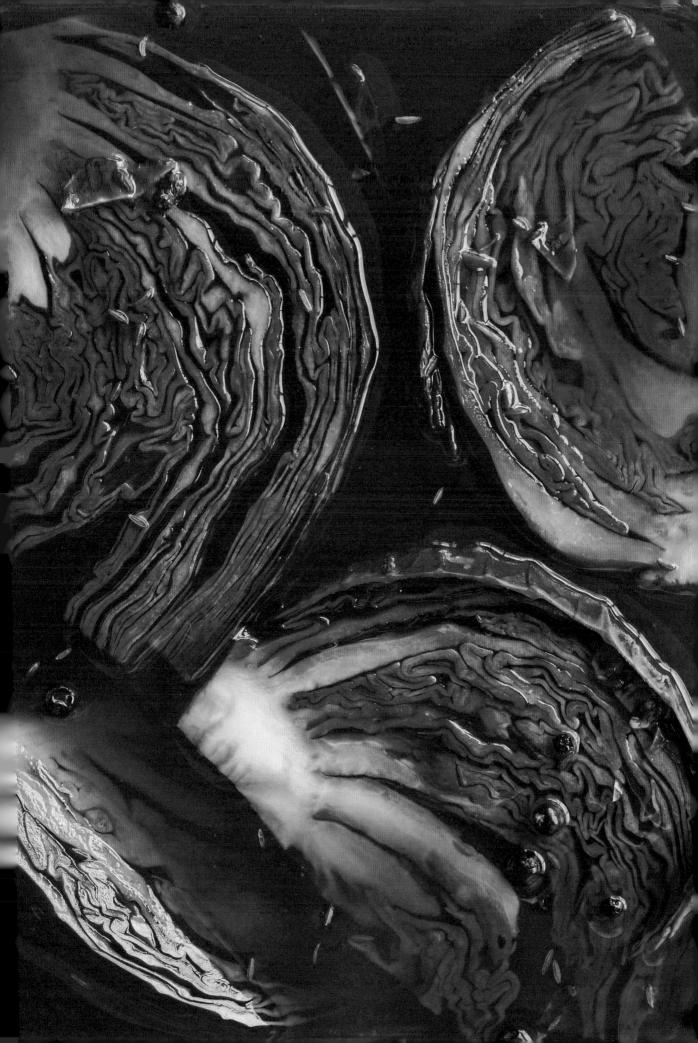

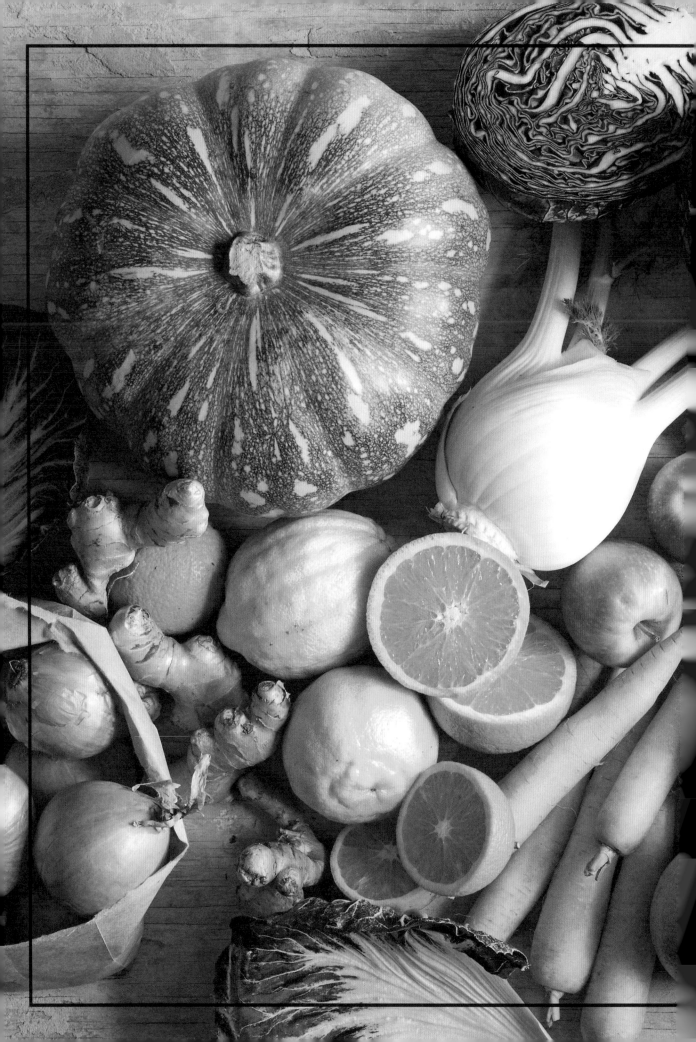

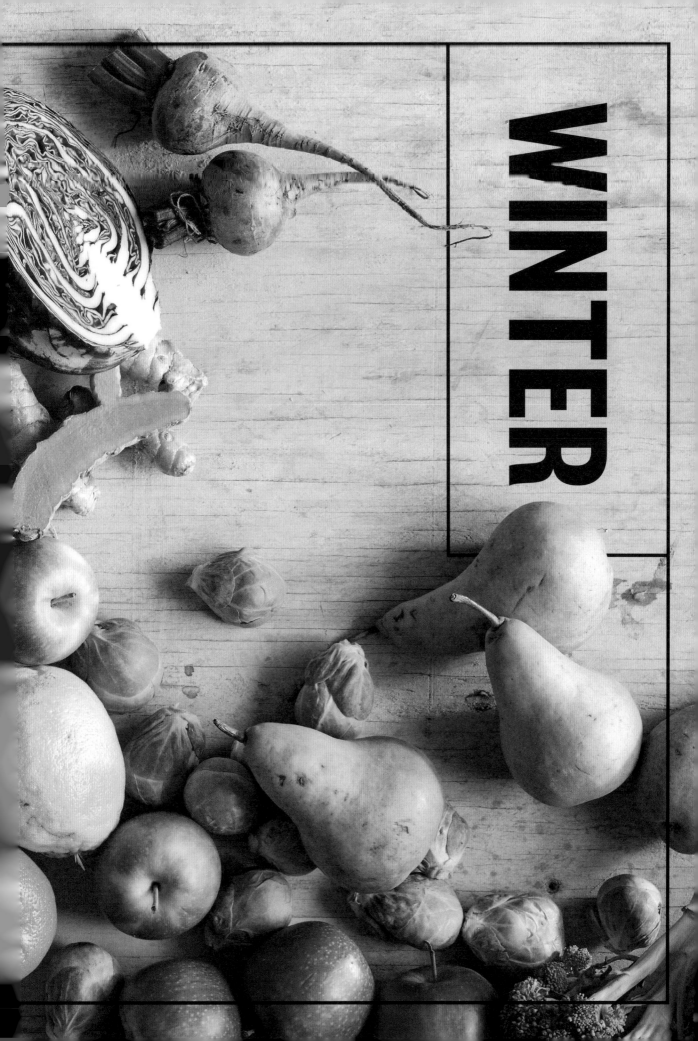

WINTER

PREPARATION TIME	SERVES
20 minutes	4

This salad is a lighter grain-free alternative to a conventional couscous salad — the cauliflower is finely chopped or grated and takes on a grain-like shape. It is very quick and simple as the ingredients require no cooking, except for toasting the hazelnuts.

At Cornersmith we make our own pomegranate molasses. You'll find the recipe in our first book, or you can buy it from specialty grocers.

CAULIFLOWER COUSCOUS WITH BROCCOLI, POMEGRANATE & TOASTED HAZELNUTS

400 g (14 oz) cauliflower, leaves removed
250 g (9 oz) broccoli
zest of ½ lemon, plus the juice of 1 lemon
2 teaspoons finely chopped preserved lemon or lime rind (or the Salt-preserved citrus skins on page 187)
2 pinches of ground cumin
¼ teaspoon ground sumac
2 pinches of chilli flakes
seeds from ½ pomegranate
40 g (1½ oz/¼ cup) toasted hazelnuts (see page 206), coarsely chopped
1 large handful of picked dill, flat-leaf (Italian) parsley and mint, torn just before serving
60 ml (2 fl oz/¼ cup) olive oil
1 tablespoon pomegranate molasses (optional)

Coarsely grate the cauliflower using a box grater, or carefully pulse it in a food processor to a couscous consistency — you don't want to chop it too small or finely, or it will be mushy. Place in a large mixing bowl.

Pick the broccoli into very small florets. Keep half the broccoli stem, peel it and slice it very thinly using a mandoline, or coarsely grate it. Add to the mixing bowl.

Add the lemon zest, preserved citrus rind, cumin, sumac and chilli flakes. Add half the pomegranate seeds, half the hazelnuts, and three-quarters of the herbs.

Season with salt, drizzle with the lemon juice and olive oil and gently combine.

Transfer to a serving bowl or large plate. Garnish with the remaining pomegranate seeds, hazelnuts and herbs, then finish with a drizzle of pomegranate molasses, if desired.

This salad is best made close to serving time.

TIP: Save your leftover broccoli stems for quick pickling (see page 162), or to use in the soba noodle dish on page 150.

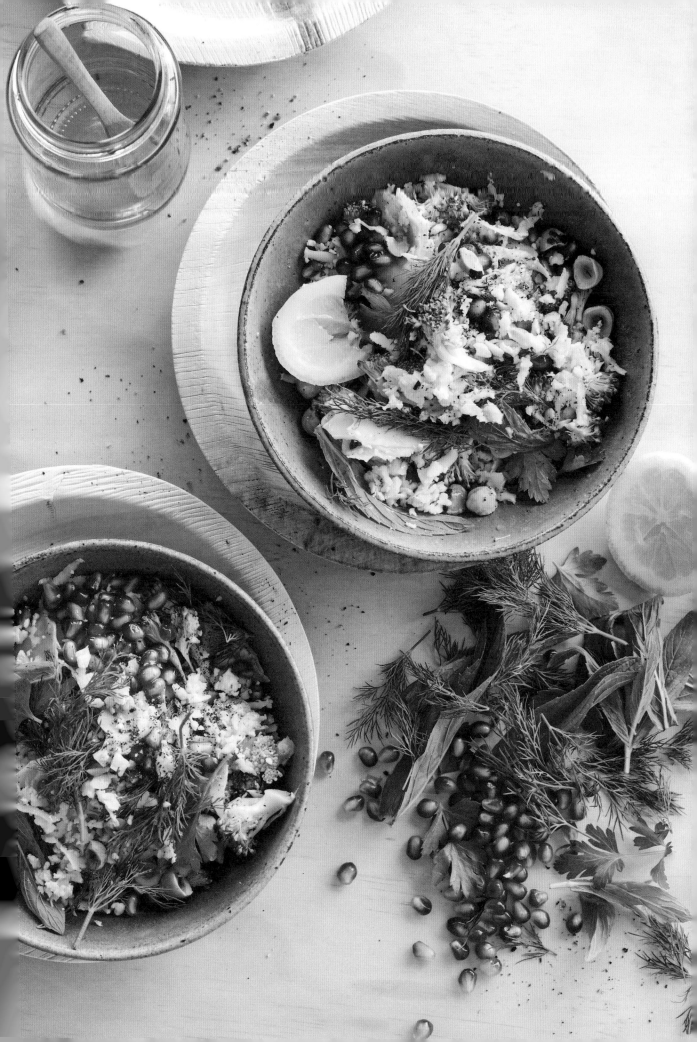

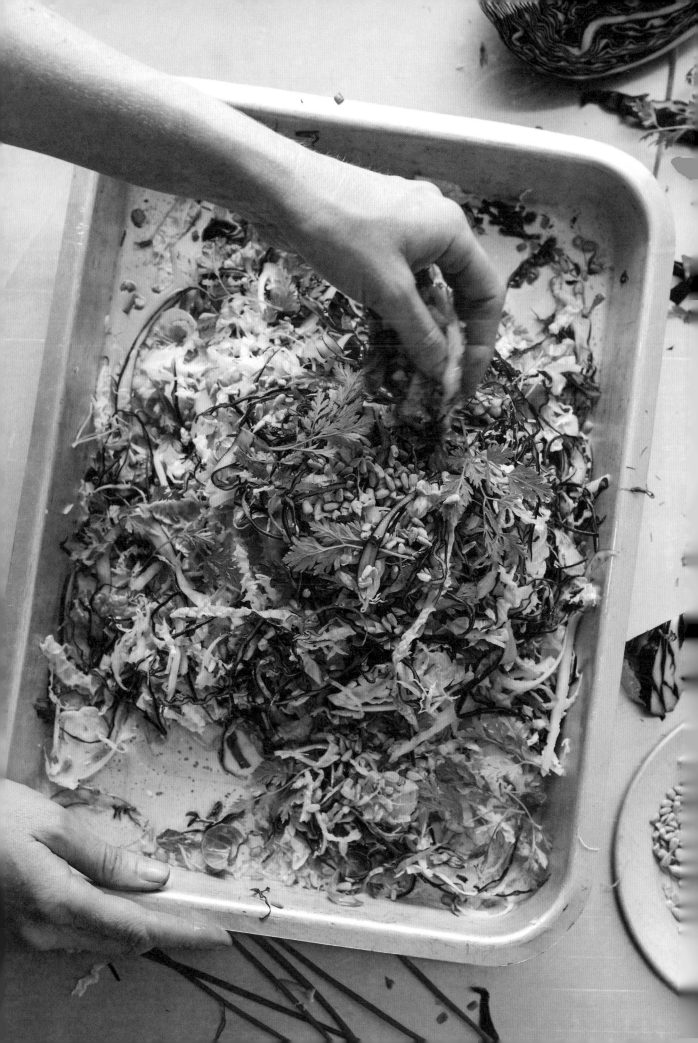

PREPARATION TIME	SERVES
20 minutes	4

Made with cabbage, wombok (a Chinese cabbage) and brussels sprouts (another member of the cabbage family), this is a very versatile salad that is great on its own, as a side, or to use in wraps and burgers. It's a lighter option to the regular mayonnaise-dressed slaws and is easy to make in bulk.

Use whatever cabbages you have available to you — white cabbage, savoy, kohlrabi — and change the herbs and seeds to use up whatever is in your fridge, pantry and garden.

You can add a soft-boiled egg or shaved parmesan to the salad if you're in the mood for something a bit richer.

THREE-CABBAGE SLAW

To make the dressing, combine the vinegars and mustard in a small jar. Season with salt and pepper and whisk together with a fork. Add the oils, put the lid on and shake well until emulsified. Set aside.

Using a mandoline, finely shave the cabbage and brussels sprouts. Place in a large mixing bowl. Thinly slice the wombok leaves and add to the bowl.

Using a mortar and pestle, roughly grind the caraway seeds and salt. Sprinkle over the slaw mixture, along with the herbs and sunflower seeds. Add the dressing and gently mix.

Place in a large bowl and serve.

TIP: The vegetables can be sliced and mixed beforehand, and the dressing could be made and kept in a jar in the fridge, but make sure the salad is dressed and assembled just before serving. Save the cabbage cores for quick pickling (see page 162) to toss through other salads. Or try the Kitchen Scrap Sauerkraut recipe on page 192, using up the remaining wombok and leftover cabbage.

1 small wedge of red cabbage
4 large brussels sprouts
3 wombok (Chinese cabbage) leaves
¼ teaspoon caraway seeds
pinch of salt
1 large handful of picked mixed herbs, such as mint, dill and chervil, finely chopped just before serving
1 tablespoon finely snipped chives
2 tablespoons toasted sunflower seeds (see page 206)

MUSTARD DRESSING
1 tablespoon aged vinegar, such as balsamic, sherry or apple balsamic
1 tablespoon apple cider vinegar
½ teaspoon dijon mustard
1½ tablespoons vegetable oil
1½ tablespoons olive oil

PREPARATION TIME	COOKING TIME	SERVES
30 minutes, plus at least 20 minutes pickling	10 minutes	4

This recipe is another staple on our cafe menu. We give this noodle salad a Cornersmith twist by adding lots of pickled stems (broccoli, broccolini, cauliflower) that would otherwise end up in the compost. You could also use the quick pickling recipe below to use up any vegetables that need eating at the end of the week. Carrots, radish and fennel work well, but just use whatever you have on hand.

Add a protein of your choice to make this salad a complete meal.

SOBA NOODLES WITH QUICK PICKLED VEGETABLES, GINGER & SESAME

½ bunch broccolini
1 small Lebanese (short) cucumber
100 g (3½ oz) slice of jap or kent pumpkin (winter squash)
200–220 g (7–8 oz) dried soba noodles
1.5 cm (⅝ inch) knob of fresh ginger, cut into very fine julienne strips
pinch of chilli flakes
1 tablespoon toasted sesame seeds (see page 206)
1 large handful of picked coriander (cilantro) sprigs
2–3 tablespoons sesame oil
1 tablespoon soy sauce (optional)
80 ml (2½ fl oz/⅓ cup) vegetable pickling liquid (from below)

QUICK PICKLING LIQUID
125 ml (4 fl oz/½ cup) apple cider vinegar
3½ tablespoons sugar
2 teaspoons salt
250 ml (9 fl oz/1 cup) very hot water

Cut off and reserve the broccolini stems, leaving about 6 cm (2½ inches) still attached. Pick the broccolini tops into small florets. Using a mandoline, very thinly slice the broccolini stems, then thinly slice the cucumber and pumpkin. Place each sliced vegetable in a separate non-reactive container.

In a small bowl, mix together all the pickling liquid ingredients, until the sugar and salt have dissolved. Pour the pickling liquid over each of the vegetables. Cover and leave to sit for at least 20 minutes, or up to 8 hours.

Near serving time, bring a large saucepan of salted water to the boil. Add the soba noodles and cook for 4 minutes, or until tender. Drain in a colander, then refresh under cold running water until they feel silky. Drain again.

Place the noodles in a large mixing bowl. Add the pickled vegetables, reserving the pickling liquid. Add the ginger strips, chilli flakes, half the sesame seeds and half the coriander and gently mix together. Now add the sesame oil and soy sauce, if using, along with 80 ml (2½ fl oz/⅓ cup) of the reserved pickling liquid. Season with salt if required.

Transfer the salad to a serving bowl, garnish with the remaining sesame seeds and coriander and serve.

TIP: Be adventurous and try doing a quick pickle with other vegetables such as cabbage, bok choy (pak choy) or wombok (Chinese cabbage).

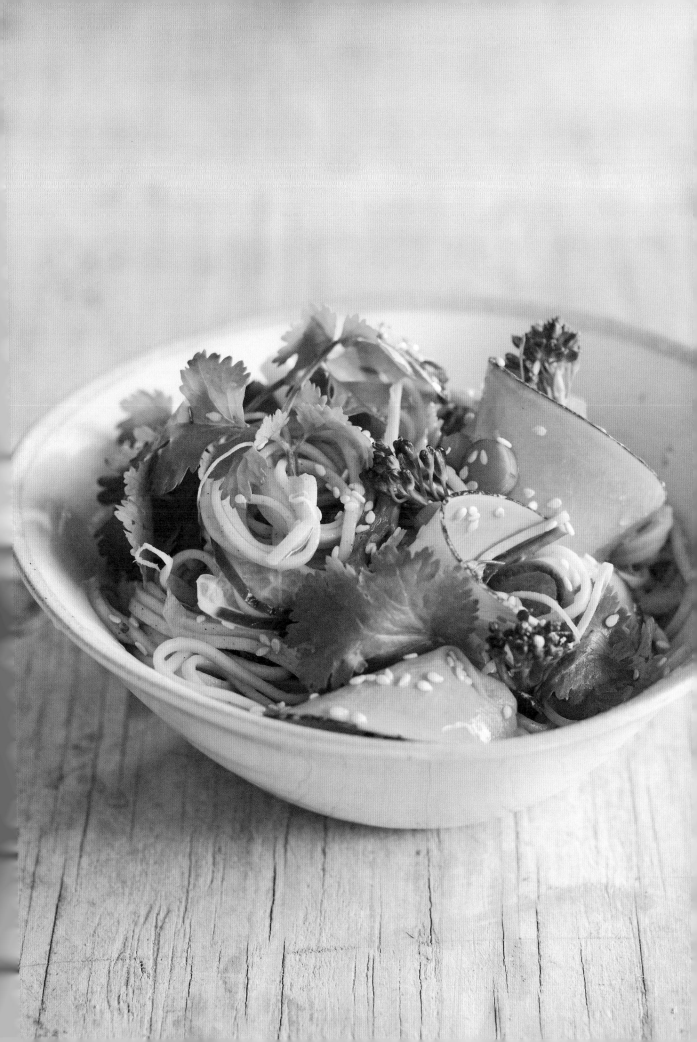

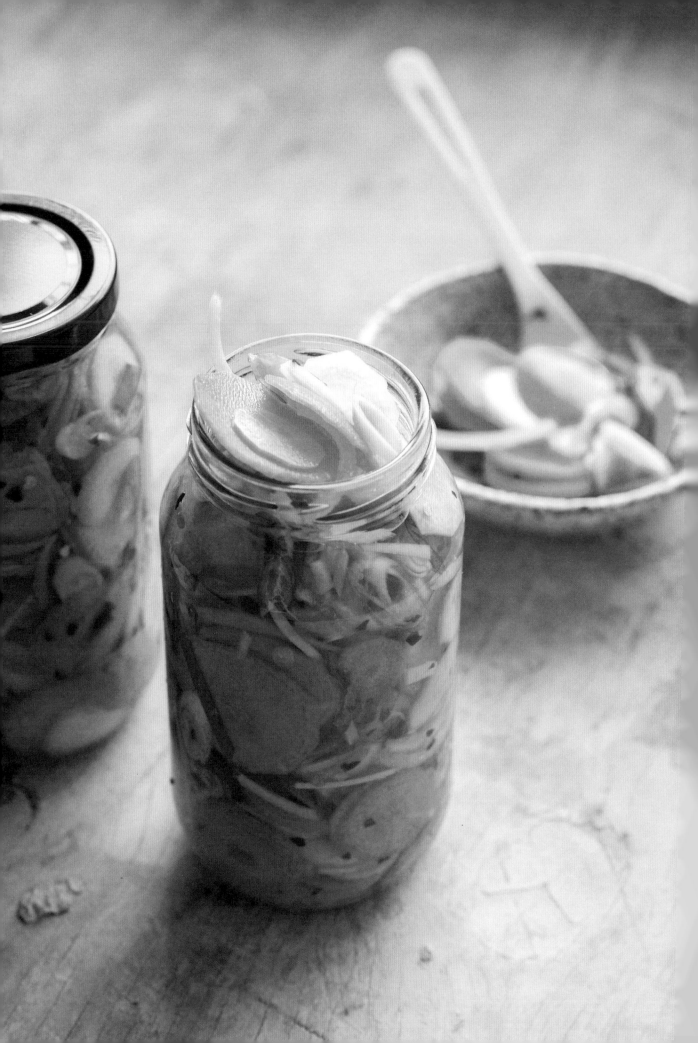

PREPARATION TIME	STORAGE	MAKES
25 minutes, plus 20 minutes sterilising, plus 15 minutes heat-processing	up to 3 months, or up to 1 year if heat-processed	2–3 x 500 ml (17 fl oz/2 cup) jars

Gingery, tangy and spicy, these carrot pickles are full of flavour. They're delicious in noodle salads, such as the soba noodle dish on page 150, or tossed through stir-fries at the end. At the cafe we also serve them on our Bibimbap (page 45). When pickling the carrots, you can also add some thinly sliced daikon, radish or choko (chayote), if you like.

PICKLED GINGER CARROTS

Make your brine by combining the vinegar, sugar, salt and water in a non-reactive, medium-sized saucepan. Place over low heat and stir to dissolve the sugar and salt. Add the chilli flakes and lemongrass, or lemon peel strips, and slowly bring to simmering point. Turn off the heat and let the brine sit so the flavours can develop.

Meanwhile, sterilise your jars and lids (see page 212).

Thinly slice the carrots, onion, spring onions and ginger, as well as any other vegetables you may be using, and mix together in a bowl.

When the jars are cool enough to handle, carefully pack the carrot mixture into them, making sure you include a bit of lemongrass or lemon peel in each jar. Bring your brine back up to the boil, then cover the carrots with the hot brine.

Remove any air bubbles by gently tapping each jar on the work surface and sliding a clean butter knife or chopstick around the inside to release any hidden air pockets. Wipe the rims of the jars with paper towel or a clean damp cloth and seal immediately.

Leave to cool on the benchtop, then store in the fridge for up to 3 months. Leave to sit for at least 2 weeks before eating. Once opened, store in the fridge and consume within 6 months.

To extend the shelf life to up to 1 year, heat-process the jars (see page 211) for 15 minutes, then store in a cool, dark place.

500 ml (17 fl oz/2 cups) rice wine vinegar (with an acidity level of 5% or more)
55 g (2 oz/¼ cup) sugar
1 teaspoon salt (see tip)
250 ml (9 fl oz/1 cup) water
1 teaspoon chilli flakes
4 lemongrass stems, white part only, cut into 4 cm (1½ inch) lengths, or 4 strips of lemon peel
500 g (1 lb 2 oz) carrots, peeled
1 small brown onion
5 spring onions (scallions)
40 g (1½ oz) knob of fresh ginger, washed well

TIP: With preserving and pickling, it is important to use 100% sea or river salt, without any additives. If your salt has added iodine, it can make the vinegar brine dark; if it contains an anti-caking agent, it can make the brine cloudy.

PREPARATION TIME	HEAT-PROCESSING	STORAGE	MAKES
30 minutes, plus 20 minutes sterilising	15 minutes	up to 2 years	2–4 x 500 ml (17 fl oz/2 cup) jars

'Canning' is what the Americans call preserving, and you should definitely give this recipe a go — you'll never want to buy beetroot in a tin again. This is one of the first pickles Alex ever made, and it's also a fun one to make with kids.

The pickled beetroot is delicious thinly sliced in salads, on burgers or with cheddar.

'CANNED' BEETROOT

1 kg (2 lb 4 oz) beetroot (beet) bulbs (trimmed weight); if your bunch has stalks and leafy tops, reserve these for pickling (see tip)
750 ml (26 fl oz/3 cups) red wine vinegar
375 ml (13 fl oz/1½ cups) water
110 g (3¾ oz/½ cup) white sugar
50 g (1¾ oz/¼ cup) brown sugar
1½ teaspoons salt

FOR EACH JAR, YOU WILL NEED:
¼ teaspoon black peppercorns
1 teaspoon dill seeds or dried dill

Sterilise your jars and lids (see page 212).

Meanwhile, wash and peel the beetroot, then slice them however you like — thin slices are great for burgers and sandwiches; wedges work well for salads and cheese plates.

Make your brine by combining the vinegar, water, all the sugar and salt in a non-reactive, medium-sized saucepan over low heat. Stir to dissolve the sugar and salt. Bring to simmering point, then turn off the heat.

When the jars are cool enough to handle, add the peppercorns and dill. Using small tongs or clean hands, carefully but tightly pack the beetroot pieces into the jars. Pour the hot brine over until they are completely covered; any leftover brine can be stored in the fridge for up to 1 month and used in salad dressings and other pickles.

Remove any air bubbles by gently tapping each jar on the work surface and sliding a clean butter knife or chopstick around the inside to release any hidden air pockets. Wipe the rims of the jars with paper towel or a clean damp cloth and seal immediately.

Heat-process the jars (see page 211) for 15 minutes, then leave to cool on the benchtop. Store in a cool, dark place for up to 2 years.

Leave to sit for at least 1 month before eating, although they will be even better after 3 months; if you've pickled whole beets, or big chunks, you'll need to let them sit longer. Once opened, store in the fridge and use within 6 months.

TIP: Beetroot stems are excellent in the quick pickles on page 162. If the leaves are in good condition, wash and dry them, then finely slice and toss through a salad, such as the baked beetroot one on page 199. At the Picklery we even collect our beetroot skins and give them to our friend Leah, who makes natural dyes for fabrics!

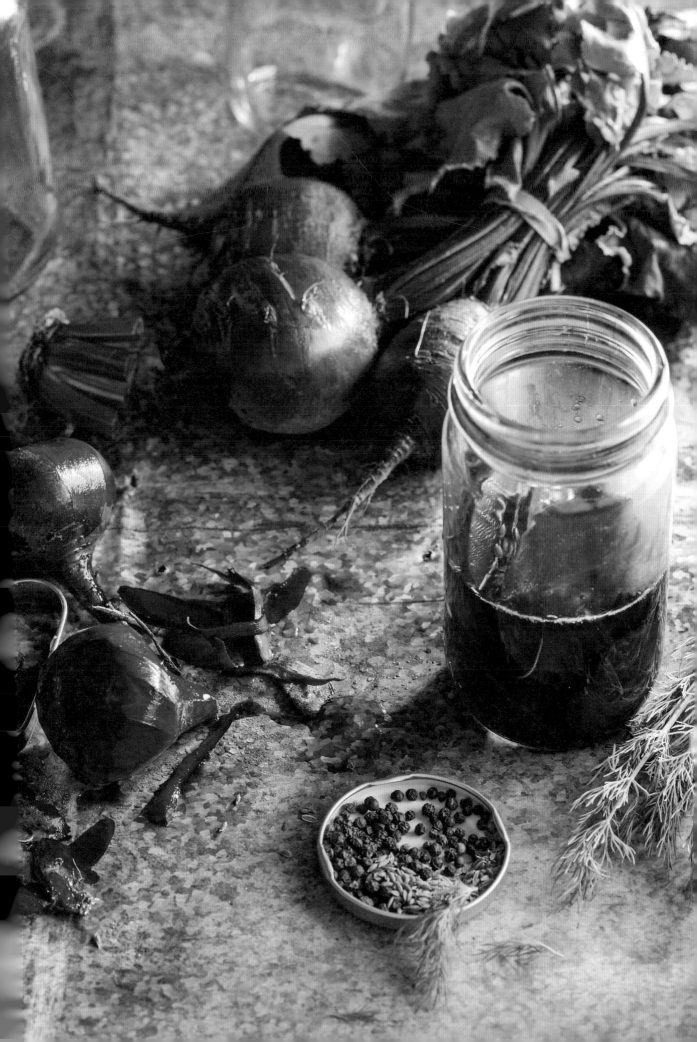

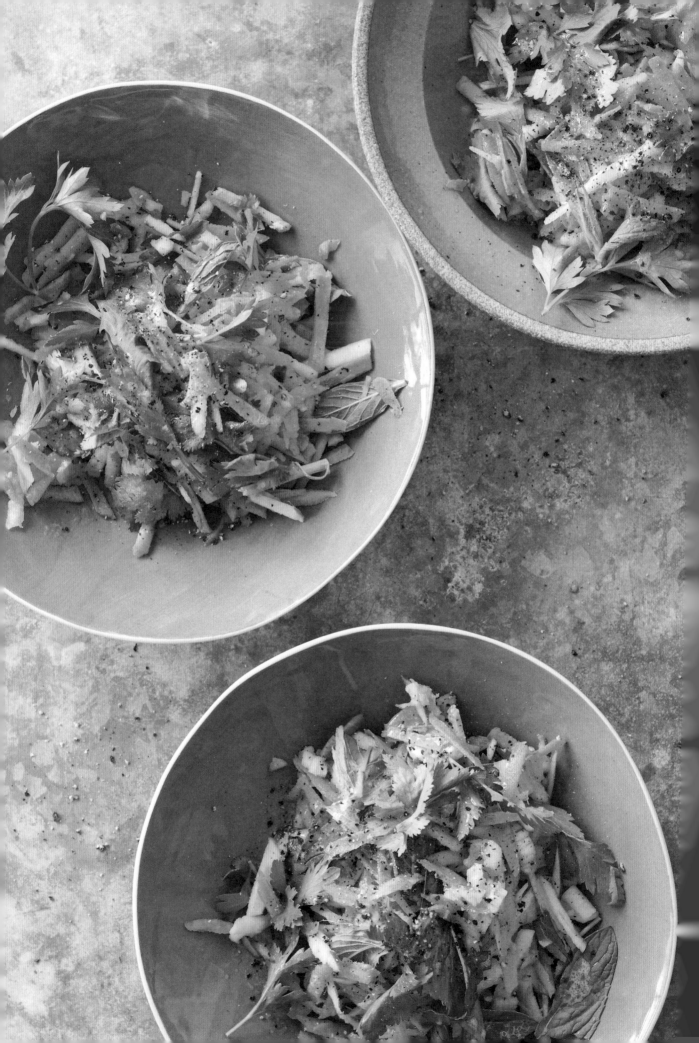

PREPARATION TIME	SERVES
10 minutes	4

This is probably the tastiest, easiest and most economical salad you can make. It's an excellent mid-week recipe as it only takes about 10 minutes to prepare, and can be made with other root vegetables such as beetroot (beet), fennel and celeriac. You can also add some toasted seeds, nuts or sprouts.

RAW CARROT & APPLE SLAW

Peel the carrots, apple and ginger. Coarsely grate the carrot and apple into a large bowl. Finely grate the ginger into the bowl, then mix the herbs through.

In a jar, combine the vinegar and mustard. Season with salt and pepper, then add the olive oil. Put the lid on and shake well until emulsified.

Toss the dressing through the carrot mixture, transfer to a serving bowl and serve.

___

TIP: If you have a little leftover grated ginger, make a quick infused vinegar by putting the grated ginger into a jar or bottle and covering with cold white wine vinegar. It's a good way to stop that last little knob of ginger going mouldy in the bottom of the fridge, and the vinegar makes an excellent base for dressings and stir-fries.

2 large carrots
1 small apple
4 cm (1½ inch) knob of fresh ginger
1 large handful of mixed picked mint, flat-leaf (Italian) parsley and coriander (cilantro) leaves
1 tablespoon apple cider vinegar
1 teaspoon dijon mustard
2 tablespoons olive oil

PREPARATION TIME	COOKING TIME	SERVES
25 minutes, plus overnight soaking	about 15 minutes	4

Inspired by flavours from the south of Spain, this hearty winter salad can definitely be served as an independent meal. The pickled onions from page 161 really make this dish — combined with the saltiness of the olives, they're a flavour sensation! If you don't happen to have any in your pantry, you can use store-bought pickled pearl or cocktail onions instead. See if you can get them in malt or apple cider vinegar, so they aren't too acidic.

You can precook the barley ahead, to reduce your preparation time on the day.

BARLEY SALAD WITH ALMONDS, OLIVES & PICKLED ONIONS

200 g (7 oz/1 cup) pearl barley, soaked in water overnight
1 teaspoon vegetable oil
6 Malt Pickled Onions (page 161), cut in half lengthways
50 g (1¾ oz/⅓ cup) pitted mixed olives, chopped
1 large handful of picked flat-leaf (Italian) parsley
2 tablespoons toasted slivered almonds (see page 206)
2 tablespoons snipped chives
1–2 pinches of smoked paprika

SMOKY BUTTERMILK DRESSING
1 tablespoon onion pickling liquid (from the Malt Pickled Onions above)
2 tablespoons buttermilk
1 teaspoon honey
1 teaspoon wholegrain mustard
¼ teaspoon smoked paprika
80 ml (2½ fl oz/⅓ cup) olive oil

Rinse the barley and drain it well. Bring a large saucepan of salted water to the boil. Add the barley, reduce the heat and simmer for 8–10 minutes, or until the grains are just cooked but still retain their shape. Remove from the heat and set aside.

Meanwhile, heat a chargrill pan or heavy cast-iron pan over medium–high heat. Add the vegetable oil and the onions to the pan, cut side down. Reduce the heat and cook for 5–8 minutes, or until the cut sides are golden brown, and show some charred marks if using a chargrill pan. Remove from the heat and leave to cool, then separate the individual onion layers or segments.

Put all the dressing ingredients, except the olive oil, in a measuring jug (or similar shaped vessel) and mix with a hand-held stick blender. With the motor running, drizzle in the oil, in a fine stream, to give a dressing with a very velvety texture. Season with salt and pepper.

Place the barley in a large mixing bowl. Add the charred onion, olives, three-quarters of the parsley and three-quarters of the almonds. Season with salt and pepper and mix together. Add the dressing and gently combine.

Pile the salad onto a platter or into a bowl. Garnish with the remaining almonds and the herbs. Sprinkle with the paprika and serve.

TIP: Instead of pearl barley, try the salad with other nutty grains such as freekeh or farro. If you don't have buttermilk, make the dressing with yoghurt and thin it out with a teaspoon of water.

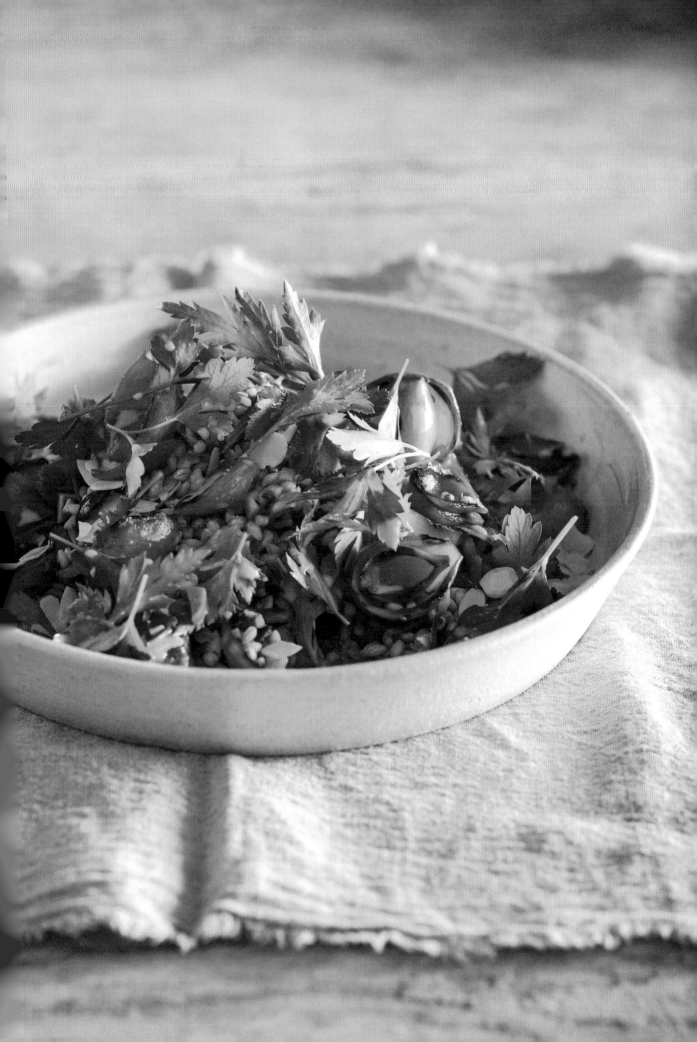

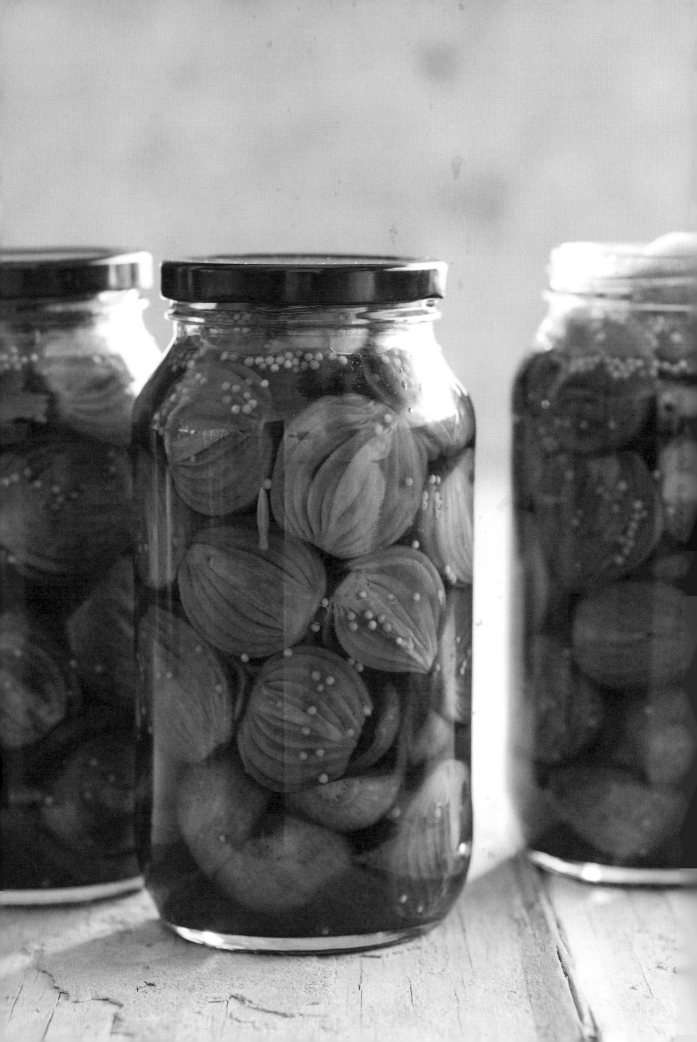

PREPARATION TIME	STORAGE	MAKES
30 minutes, plus overnight salting, plus 20 minutes sterilising	up to 1 year	3–4 x 500 ml (17 fl oz/2 cup) jars

We've made so many different versions of pickled onions over the years. These ones are rich in colour and flavour, and make you think instantly about eating cheddar. Pickled onions are a good option in salads to add some sweetness and bite, rather than raw onions, which can be a bit intense. Unusually, there is no water in this pickling brine, as the onions have enough water in them already.

MALT PICKLED ONIONS

Plunge the whole onions in boiling water for 30 seconds, then run under cold water. Peel off the skins. Leave small onions whole, and cut larger ones in half or quarters.

Place the onions in a large non-reactive bowl. Sprinkle with the salt and leave in the fridge overnight. This will draw out any excess moisture and keep your onions crisp.

The next day, make your pickling brine by combining the vinegar, sugar, ginger and all the spices in a non-reactive, medium-sized saucepan over low heat. Stir to dissolve the sugar, bring to simmering point, then turn off the heat and let the flavours infuse the vinegar.

Meanwhile, sterilise your jars and lids (see page 212).

When the jars are cool enough to handle, rinse your onions under cold water to remove the salt, then drain well. Pack the onions firmly into the jars, being sure to leave 1 cm (½ inch) space at the top.

Bring your brine back up to the heat — it needs to be very hot before you pour it over the onions.

Pour the hot vinegar brine over the onions, evenly distributing the spices among the jars. Make sure the onions are completely submerged.

Remove any air bubbles by gently tapping each jar on the benchtop and sliding a clean butter knife or chopstick around the inside to release any hidden air pockets. Wipe the rims with paper towel and seal immediately.

Leave to cool on the benchtop, then store in a cool, dark place for up to 1 year. The onions can be eaten after 4–6 weeks, but will be even better after 3 months. Once opened, store in the fridge and use within 6 months.

1 kg (2 lb 4 oz) small brown onions
3 tablespoons pure salt
750 ml (26 fl oz/3 cups) malt vinegar
300 g (10½ oz/1½ cups) brown sugar
4 slices well-washed fresh ginger
6 star anise
12 cloves
12 allpsice berries
3 teaspoons yellow mustard seeds
¼ teaspoon cayenne pepper

TIP: For lighter, tangier pickled onions, use apple cider vinegar instead of malt vinegar. Use 55 g (2 oz/¼ cup) white sugar and 50 g (1¾ oz/¼ cup) brown sugar. Leave out the star anise, cloves and cayenne pepper, and add 2 bay leaves to each jar with the ginger and allspice.

PREPARATION TIME	STORAGE	MAKES
15 minutes, plus 20 minutes cooling	up to 2 weeks	1 x 500 ml (17 fl oz/2 cup) container

Quick pickling is a great way to use up any vegetables in the fridge at the end of the week, as well as those leftover vegie stems — cauliflower, beetroot, broccoli and kale stems all make really delicious pickles! And it's so simple: no need to worry about sterilising jars and lids sealing.

These pickles need to be kept in the fridge, and will last for about 2 weeks in an airtight jar or sealed container.

If you have any leftover brine from the bottom of other jars of pickles, you can gently heat it up in a small saucepan and use it for quick-pickling, following the same method below.

QUICK KITCHEN-SCRAP PICKLE

125 ml (4 fl oz/½ cup) white wine vinegar, rice wine vinegar, apple cider vinegar or red wine vinegar
250 ml (9 fl oz/1 cup) very hot water
75 g (2½ oz/⅓ cup) sugar
2 teaspoons salt
1 cup sliced vegetables of your choice
1 teaspoon spices of your choice, or a few slices of fresh ginger, chilli or a bay leaf

To make the brine, combine the vinegar, hot water, sugar and salt in a jug. Stir until the sugar and salt have dissolved.

Add your thinly sliced vegetables and your spices to a non-reactive container. Mix together well.

Pour the hot brine over the vegetables and leave to sit for at least 20 minutes.

Once cooled, cover and store in the fridge. The pickles will last for up to 2 weeks.

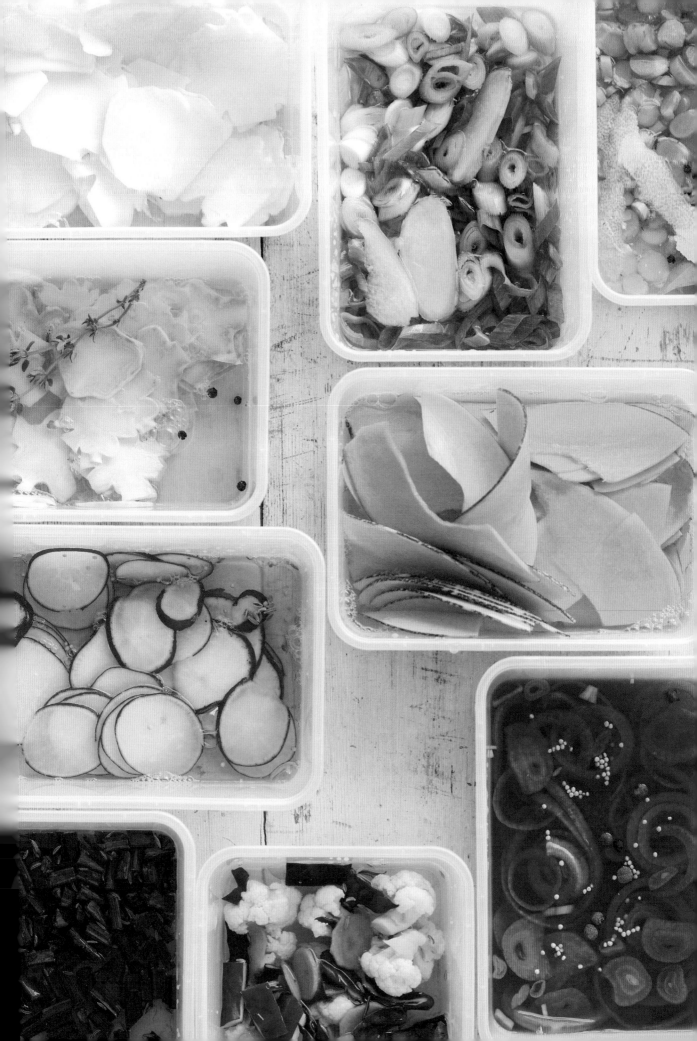

FLAVOURED VINEGARS

Flavouring vinegars is so easy, and a good way to use up half bunches of herbs, the knob of ginger left in the bottom of your fridge, the peel from a lemon when you've only used its juice, and so on. Flavoured vinegars are great to have on hand for deliciously easy salad dressings, quick pickling, dipping sauces and marinades. They also look so pretty in bottles and they make lovely gifts.

Simply put your ingredients in a sterilised jar or bottle and cover with white wine vinegar, rice wine vinegar, apple cider vinegar or red wine vinegar. Leave to infuse for 3–4 weeks. During this time, keep tasting the vinegar, and one day you'll know it's ready; it's really up to you how long you leave it. Strain, then return the flavoured vinegar to the bottle and store it in the cupboard or fridge. Your vinegar will last for up to 2 years, but just remember that the flavour will deteriorate over time.

You don't need to buy the most expensive vinegar on the shelf for infusing vinegars, but you do want a vinegar that has a nice soft flavour and isn't too acidic. Never use straight-up white vinegar for these recipes, as its astringency will overpower the flavour of your aromatic ingredients.

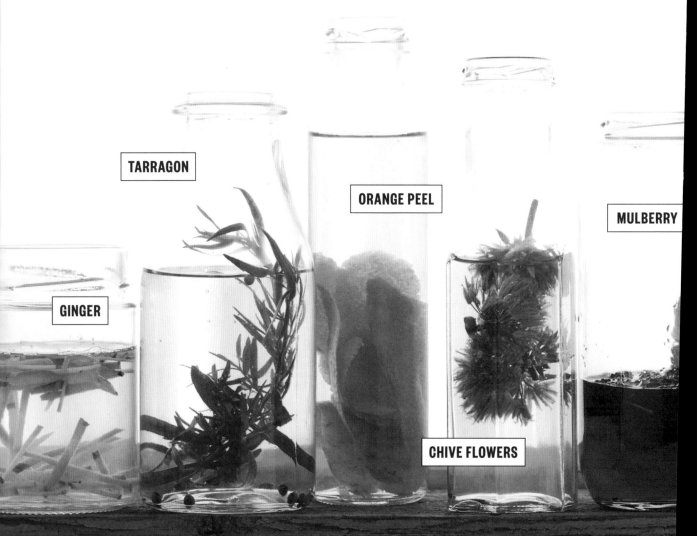

TARRAGON

ORANGE PEEL

MULBERRY

GINGER

CHIVE FLOWERS

Always match your ingredients to your vinegar. So herbs would be lovely with white wine vinegar; chillies, lemongrass and garlic would work well with rice wine vinegar; and fruits would pair nicely with apple cider vinegar.

We've given you single flavour ideas over the page, but you can also experiment with mixing other favourite ingredients together as well — rosemary, garlic and lemon peel; ginger, lime and chilli; mulberry, orange and peppercorn.

If you want to make your infused vinegar more of a ready-made salad dressing base, you can add a small amount of sugar and salt (to taste) into the bottom of your jar with your other ingredients. For 250 ml (9 fl oz/1 cup) vinegar, start with ½ teaspoon of both salt and sugar, let the flavours develop for a few weeks, and then add more seasoning if needed.

We always use cold vinegar to infuse flavour. This helps keep the good properties of raw vinegars alive, but it will take a little longer to infuse in the colder months. You can use warmed vinegar to speed up the process.

This is such an easy and satisfying preserving technique, so get started!

Over the page are a few seasonal ideas to help get you on your way.

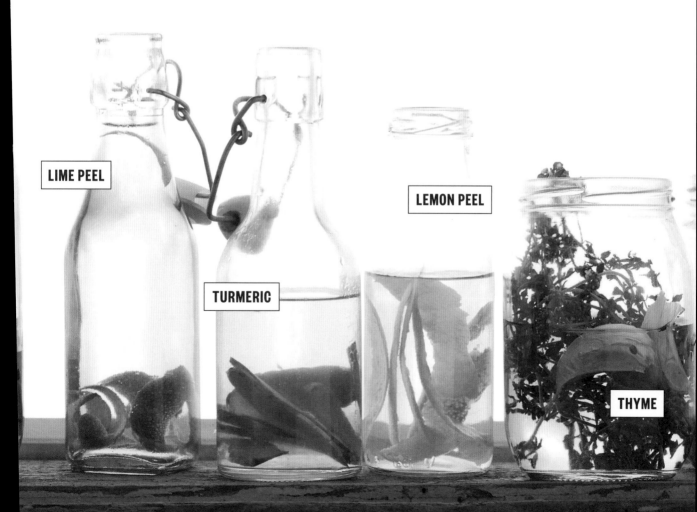

LIME PEEL

TURMERIC

LEMON PEEL

THYME

SPRING

HERB VINEGAR
Use 3 heaped tablespoons of fresh herbs, such as sage, rosemary, parsley, chives, bay, thyme, oregano and a few white peppercorns. You can either do a single flavour, or a mixed herb combination. Place in a small sterilised glass jar or bottle. Cover with 250 ml (9 fl oz/1 cup) cold apple cider vinegar or white wine vinegar and leave to infuse for 3–4 weeks. Strain, then pour the vinegar back into the bottle. Seal and store in the cupboard.

GARLIC VINEGAR
Use 2 blanched garlic cloves, skin left on, lightly bruised or bashed. Place in a small sterilised glass jar or bottle. Cover with 250 ml (9 fl oz/1 cup) cold apple cider vinegar or white wine vinegar and leave to infuse for 3–4 weeks. Strain, then pour the vinegar back into the bottle. Seal and store in the cupboard.

NASTURTIUM VINEGAR
Place 4 small nasturtium leaves, a few nasturtium flowers and some nasturtium capers (the young green unripe nasturtium seed pods) in a small sterilised glass jar or bottle. Add 1 garlic clove, ½ teaspoon sugar, ½ teaspoon salt and a few black peppercorns. Cover with 250 ml (9 fl oz/1 cup) cold apple cider vinegar or white wine vinegar and leave to infuse for 3–4 weeks. Strain, then pour the vinegar back into the bottle. Seal and store in the cupboard.

FENNEL VINEGAR & FENNEL HONEY
We pick the flowers, seeds and fronds from the fennel that grows wild along the river to make flavoured vinegars and infused honey; we also use the flowers and seeds in our vegetable pickles. Place a few fennel flower heads in a small sterilised glass jar or bottle. Cover with 250 ml (9 fl oz/1 cup) cold apple cider vinegar, white wine vinegar or honey and leave to infuse for 3–4 weeks. Strain, then pour the vinegar or honey back into the bottle. Seal and store in the cupboard.

SUMMER

MULBERRY VINEGAR
Mash 3 tablespoons fresh mulberries and 1 tablespoon of sugar together in a bowl. Scoop the mixture into a small sterilised glass jar or bottle and cover with 250 ml (9 fl oz/1 cup) cold apple cider vinegar or red wine vinegar. Seal and leave to infuse for 1–2 weeks on the benchtop (or in the fridge if the weather is very hot), then strain and discard the mulberry flesh. Pour the vinegar back into the bottle, then seal and store in the fridge. This vinegar turns a lovely colour and is a great base for salad dressings.

CHILLI VINEGAR
Pierce 2–3 chillies with a sharp knife. Put the chillies in a small sterilised glass jar or bottle and cover with 250 ml (9 fl oz/1 cup) cold white wine vinegar or rice wine vinegar. Seal and leave to infuse for 2–4 weeks, depending on how hot you'd like it! Strain, then pour the vinegar back into the bottle. Seal and store in the cupboard. The chillies will be well preserved and can be added to sauces or marinades; they will keep in an airtight container in the fridge for a week or so.

STONE FRUIT KERNEL VINEGAR
Stone fruit kernels have a lot of amazing flavour in them. They taste fruity and almondy and when they're covered in raw apple cider vinegar the flavour really comes out. After you've eaten peaches or prunes or made plum chutney make sure you keep some of the kernels. Put 4–6 stone fruit kernels in a clean jar and cover with 250 ml (9 fl oz/1 cup) cold apple cider vinegar. Leave to infuse for a few weeks, then strain and discard the kernels. Pour the vinegar back into the bottle, then seal and store in the fridge.

AUTUMN

MULLED VINEGAR

Put 1 star anise, 4 peppercorns, 2 cloves and 1 cinnamon stick or bay leaf in a small sterilised glass jar. Cover with 250 ml (9 fl oz/ 1 cup) warm red wine vinegar. Seal and leave to infuse for 2–4 weeks, then strain and discard the spices. Pour the vinegar back into the bottle, then seal and store in the cupboard. This mulled vinegar is great mixed with olive oil to dress beetroot (beets), and in marinades for meats.

PERSIMMON VINEGAR

If you have a very overripe persimmon, scoop the flesh into a small sterilised glass jar or bottle and cover with 250 ml (9 fl oz/1 cup) cold white wine vinegar or apple cider vinegar. Seal and leave to infuse for 1–2 weeks (or in the fridge if the weather is very hot). Strain and discard the persimmon flesh, then pour the vinegar back into the bottle. Seal and store in the fridge. This vinegar goes a lovely orange colour and is a great base for salad dressings.

FIRE TONIC

To get your immune system ready for winter, put 1 chilli, a few slices of fresh ginger, 1 slice of fresh turmeric, 1 tablespoon diced onion, and a few black peppercorns into a small sterilised jar or bottle. Cover with 250 ml (9 fl oz/1 cup) cold raw unfiltered apple cider vinegar (with the 'mother' culture), then seal. You don't need to strain this vinegar. A teaspoon of this one every day will help keep the winter colds at bay.

WINTER

LEMON / ORANGE / LIME VINEGAR

Peel one piece of citrus fruit, avoiding as much of the bitter white pith as you can. Put the peel in a small sterilised glass jar or bottle and cover with 250 ml (9 fl oz/1 cup) cold white wine vinegar or apple cider vinegar. Seal and leave to infuse for 3–4 weeks, then strain and discard the peel. Pour the vinegar back into the bottle, then seal and store in the cupboard. (See page 27 for a salad dressing recipe.)

GINGER / TURMERIC VINEGAR

Peel and grate a 40 g (1½ oz) knob of fresh ginger or turmeric and place in a small sterilised glass jar or bottle. Add ½ teaspoon salt and 5 black peppercorns. Cover with 250 ml (9 fl oz/1 cup) cold white wine vinegar or apple cider vinegar. Seal and leave to infuse for 3–4 weeks, then strain. Pour the vinegar back into the bottle, then seal and store in the cupboard.

HORSERADISH VINEGAR

Peel and grate a 30 g (1 oz) knob of fresh horseradish. Place in a small sterilised glass jar or bottle with 1 tablespoon thinly sliced chives, 1 thinly sliced French shallot, 6 white peppercorns, 1 teaspoon sugar and ½ teaspoon salt. Cover with 250 ml (9 fl oz/ 1 cup) cold apple cider vinegar or white wine vinegar. Seal and leave to infuse on the benchtop for 3–4 weeks. Then strain the vinegar out, discard the horseradish mixture and pour into a clean sterilised bottle. Store in the cupboard.

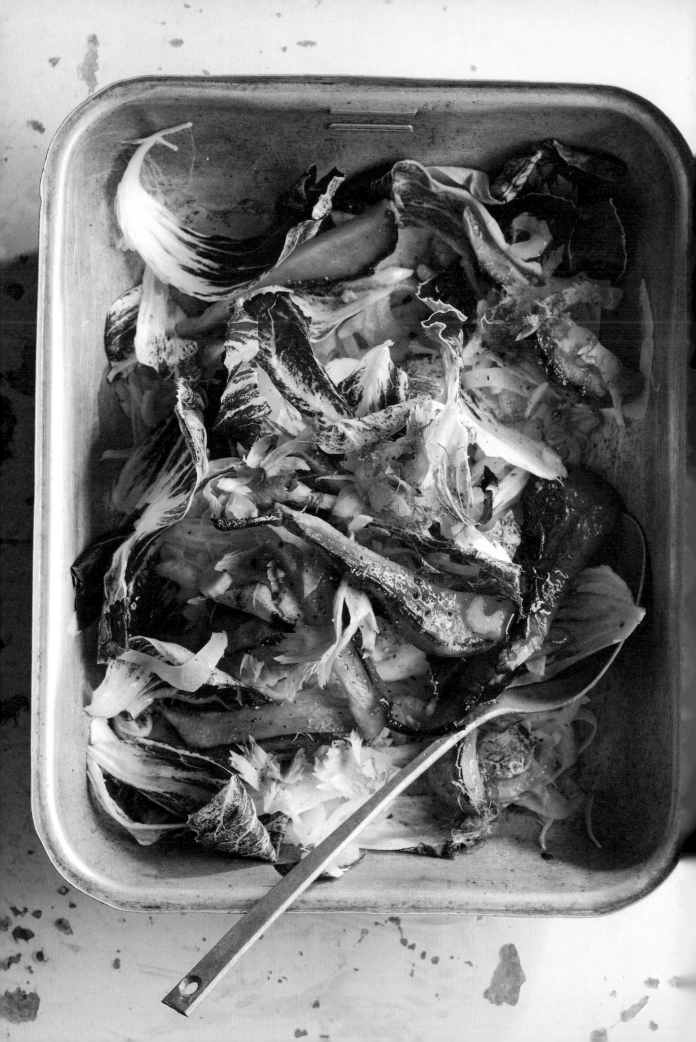

PREPARATION TIME	COOKING TIME	SERVES
20 minutes	about 30 minutes	4

Many wintery leaves are on the bitter end of the flavour spectrum. In our experience, some people are a little prejudiced against bitter flavours, so at our cafes we try to keep integrating these into our winter menus, by counteracting the bitterness with an element of sweetness. This is how the idea for this salad came together. It has a great balance of wintery bitter leaves, sweetness from the pears and the anise flavour of the fennel. Try it with a dollop of ricotta.

BITTER WINTER LEAVES WITH FENNEL & ROASTED PEAR

Preheat the oven to 175°C (350°F). Line a small baking tray, just large enough to fit all the pear wedges, with baking paper.

Make a syrup for the pears by combining the lemon juice, sugar, honey, ginger and salt in a bowl and whisking until the sugar has dissolved. Add the pear wedges and coat them well. Place the pear wedges on the lined baking tray, drizzle with the syrup and bake for about 25 minutes, or until golden brown.

Meanwhile, pick the green fronds and leaves from the fennel and celery and reserve as garnishes. Thinly shave the fennel bulb, using a mandoline. Place in a large mixing bowl and toss the lemon juice through, so the fennel doesn't discolour. Thinly slice the celery and add to the bowl.

Trim the base of the radicchio, then tear the leaves into bite-sized pieces. Add to the fennel mixture with the chilli flakes, season with salt and pepper and gently toss to combine.

Place the leaves on a large serving plate or in a bowl and arrange the roasted pear wedges on top. Drizzle a bit of the pear roasting syrup over the leaves. Garnish with the reserved celery leaves and fennel fronds, drizzle with the olive oil and serve.

½ fennel bulb, with some
    green fronds attached
3 celery stalks, with some
    green leaves attached
juice of ½ lemon
6−8 radicchio leaves, ends
    trimmed, torn
pinch of chilli flakes
2 tablespoons olive oil

FOR THE ROASTED PEARS
juice of ½ lemon
1 tablespoon caster (superfine)
    sugar
2 teaspoons honey
¼ teaspoon grated fresh ginger
pinch of salt
1 large pear, beurre bosc
    if possible, cored and cut
    into 8 wedges

TIP: All our salads are best made just before serving and eaten immediately. Most of them — except the leaf-based ones — will be fine for leftovers the next day, but won't look or taste their finest. You can make many of the elements ahead, store them separately, and assemble and dress just before serving.

PREPARATION TIME	COOKING TIME	SERVES
30 minutes, plus 15 minutes steaming	10 minutes	4

Roasting couscous deepens the flavour of the grain in this delicious winter salad. As there's so much citrus around at this time of year, make this salad a nourishing winter staple. Feel free to add other herbs and nuts, and experiment with different citrus fruits such as blood orange, pomelo and limes.

ROASTED COUSCOUS & CITRUS SALAD WITH TURMERIC DRESSING

1 tablespoon capers, chopped
   (or use whole baby capers)
1 pink grapefruit, filleted into
   segments
1 orange, filleted into segments
1 large handful of mixed picked
   flat-leaf (Italian) parsley
   and mint leaves, torn just
   before serving
1 heaped tablespoon toasted
   almonds (see page 206),
   roughly chopped
1 tablespoon olive oil

FOR THE COUSCOUS
60 ml (2 fl oz/¼ cup) olive oil
200 g (7 oz/1 cup) couscous
¼ teaspoon salt
½ teaspoon ground cumin
zest of 2 oranges, and the juice
   of 3 oranges
zest and juice of 1 lemon
½ teaspoon harissa paste

TURMERIC DRESSING
1 tablespoon Turmeric Vinegar
   (page 167)
2 tablespoons natural
   unsweetened yoghurt
½ garlic clove, crushed
pinch of ground cumin

To prepare the couscous, warm the olive oil in a large heavy-based saucepan over medium heat. Add the couscous and salt. Stir constantly for about 5 minutes, until the couscous starts colouring.

Add the cumin and all the citrus zest. Cook, stirring constantly, until the spices become fragrant.

Add the harissa, stir for another minute, then stir in all the citrus juice and 50 ml (1¾ fl oz) water.

Bring back up to a simmer for 2–3 minutes, then put the lid on and turn off the heat. Leave to steam, covered, for about 10–15 minutes.

Meanwhile, combine all the dressing ingredients in a small bowl. Mix until smooth, adding salt to taste.

Loosen the cooled couscous with a fork, then place in a large mixing bowl. Add the capers, citrus segments and most of the herbs. Carefully mix to combine, then check the seasoning.

Transfer to a salad bowl or large plates. Pour the dressing over and garnish with the remaining herbs and the almonds. Drizzle with the olive oil and serve.

TIP: The turmeric vinegar is very easy to make, but needs to be prepared in advance (see page 167). If you don't have any, you can add 1–2 pinches of ground turmeric into apple cider vinegar and use that in your dressing. All the salad elements can be prepared ahead and stored separately. Assemble and dress the salad just before serving.

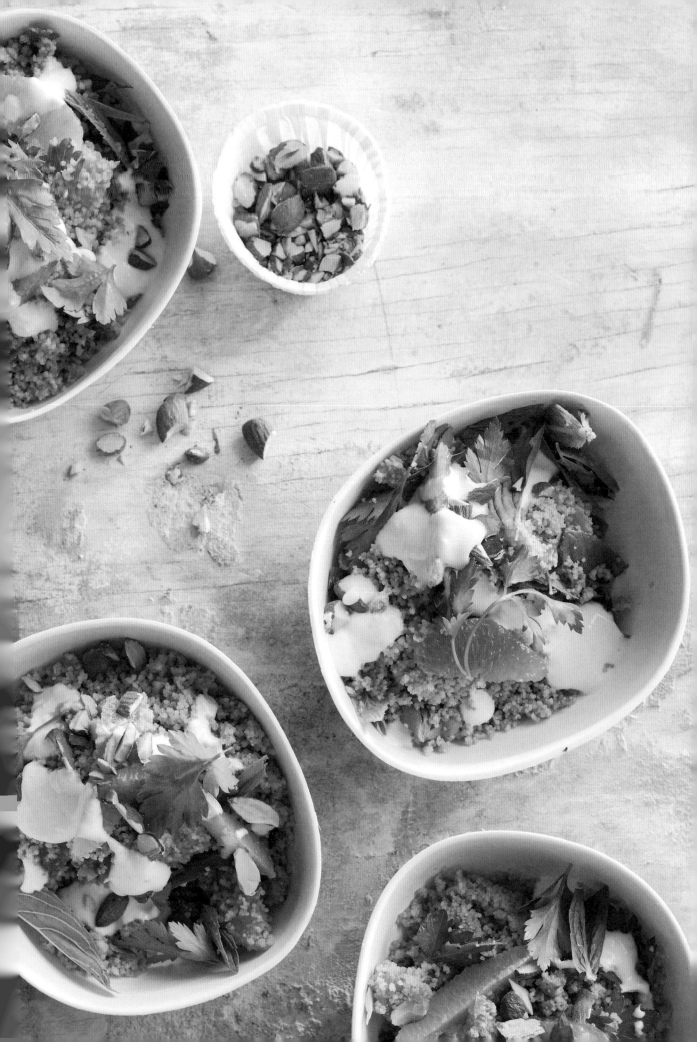

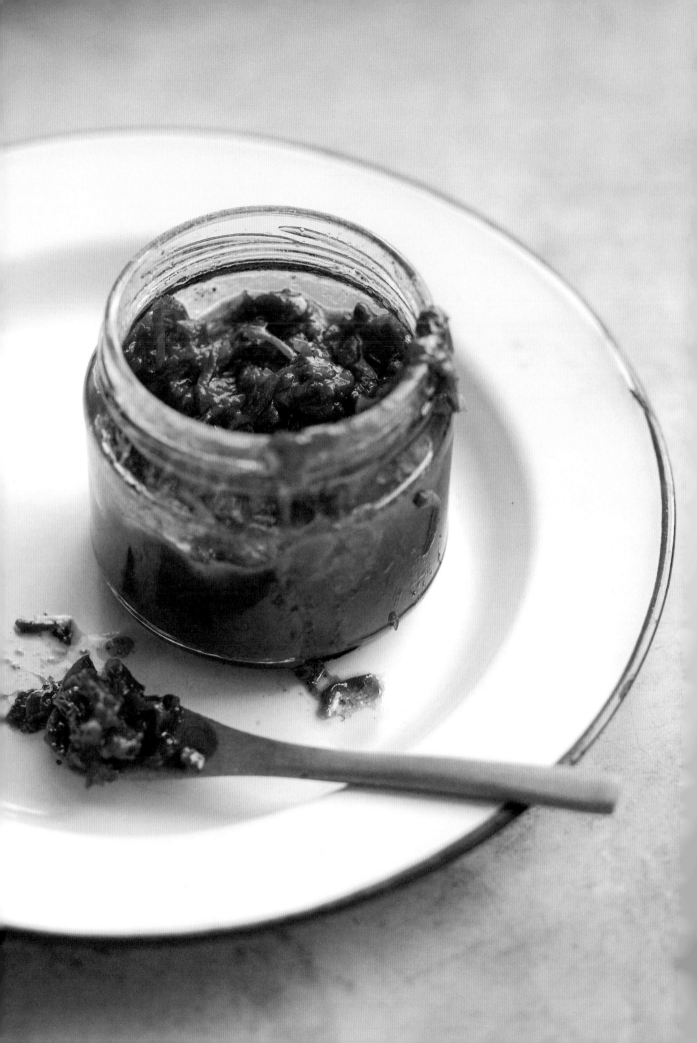

PREPARATION TIME	COOKING TIME	STORAGE	MAKES
40 minutes, plus 20 minutes sterilising, plus 10 minutes heat-processing (optional)	about 2¼ hours	up to 1 year, or up to 2 years if heat-processed	3–4 x 300 ml (10½ fl oz) jars

Sticky and very rich in flavour, this relish is inspired by the worcestershire sauce that we make at the Picklery. You need to cook this one for a long time to get the right consistency and colour, but it's well worth it. Make sure you sauté the onion down in batches, or you'll end up with a soupy pot of oniony liquid.

Serve this relish on a ploughman's plate or a toasted sandwich, or use a few tablespoons in a marinade for meats.

STICKY ONION WORCESTERSHIRE RELISH

Find yourself a large, non-reactive saucepan — for even evaporation, it's better to use a wider and more shallow pan for this recipe than a stockpot.

Heat the oil in the saucepan over medium heat. Add half the onion and half the salt. Slowly soften for about 15 minutes, stirring often, until the onion is starting to collapse. Now stir in the remaining onion and cook, stirring often, for about 20 minutes, until all the onion is evenly cooked, and the liquid has evaporated — you don't want the onions stewing in their own juices.

Stir in all the ground spices and ginger and gently cook for about 5 minutes, until fragrant, stirring constantly. Add the vinegar, water, molasses, sugar, lemon zest, lemon juice and the remaining salt, stirring to dissolve the sugar.

Gently cook over low heat for up to 1½ hours, until the relish is glossy and sticky, stirring often to prevent sticking. When your onion relish is ready there will be no vinegar pooling on the surface, and you should be able to run your spoon through the centre and see the bottom of the pan.

Meanwhile, sterilise your jars and lids (see page 212).

Carefully fill the hot jars with the hot relish. Remove any air bubbles by sliding a clean butter knife or chopstick around the inside to release any hidden air pockets. Wipe the rims of the jars with paper towel or a clean damp cloth and seal immediately.

Cool on the benchtop, then store in a cool, dark place for up to 1 year. Try to leave for at least 1 month before eating. To extend the shelf life to 2 years, heat-process the jars (see page 211) for 10 minutes. Once opened, store in the fridge and use within 6 months.

80 ml (2½ fl oz/⅓ cup) olive or vegetable oil
1.5 kg (3 lb 5 oz) onions, thinly sliced
1 tablespoon salt
½ teaspoon ground cloves
½ teaspoon ground allspice
½ teaspoon ground star anise
½ teaspoon ground black pepper
¼ teaspoon cayenne pepper
½ teaspoon ground cinnamon
½ teaspoon freshly grated nutmeg
40 g (1½ oz) grated fresh ginger
750 ml (26 fl oz/3 cups) malt vinegar
250 ml (9 fl oz/1 cup) water
115 g (4 oz/⅓ cup) molasses
250 g (9 oz/1¼ cups) brown sugar
zest and juice of 1 lemon

PREPARATION TIME	COOKING TIME	SERVES
20 minutes, plus 15 minutes soaking	35 minutes, plus 10 minutes resting	4

Leek is such an underrated vegetable, often only used for stocks and soups. Braising turns it into a sweet, rich and delicious dish, which is especially lovely at this time of the year.

BRAISED LEEKS WITH CRESS, CHOPPED EGG & MUSTARD DRESSING

4 small leeks
pinch of freshly grated nutmeg
2–3 thyme sprigs
50 g (1¾ oz) butter, diced
100 ml (3½ fl oz) olive oil

MUSTARD DRESSING
1–2 tablespoons braising liquid, from the leeks
2 teaspoons red wine vinegar
1 teaspoon dijon mustard
60 ml (2 fl oz/¼ cup) olive oil

TO FINISH
2 hard-boiled eggs, shelled and finely chopped
1½ tablespoons snipped chives
1 handful of picked watercress sprigs

Trim the root end from the leeks, then soak the leeks in water for 10–15 minutes to wash off any grit.

Meanwhile, preheat the oven to 180°C (350°F).

Cut the leeks in half lengthways. Line a baking dish with a piece of foil large enough to fold into a parcel around the leeks. Place a sheet of baking paper on the foil.

Place the leeks on the baking paper. Season with salt and pepper, sprinkle with the nutmeg, and top with the thyme sprigs and butter cubes. Drizzle with the olive oil and 150 ml (5 fl oz) water, then close the foil around the leeks, into a parcel.

Bake for 30–35 minutes, or until just cooked through. Remove from the oven and let the leeks sit in the foil parcel for about 10 minutes to absorb the flavours.

Open the parcel and let the leeks cool down. Reserve the braising juices, and pour 1–2 tablespoons of the braising juices into a screw-top jar for the vinaigrette. Add the vinegar and mustard and combine with a small whisk or fork. Add the olive oil, put the lid on and shake well. Season to taste with salt and pepper.

In a small bowl, gently mix together the chopped eggs, chives and watercress.

Arrange the warm leeks on a platter. Drizzle with half the dressing, top with the watercress and egg mixture, then finish with the remaining dressing. Serve warm.

The leeks can be braised a day ahead, then gently warmed in the oven before assembling the salad for serving.

TIP: Keep the leftover braising liquid from the leeks to add to your next potato and leek soup. The braising liquid can be frozen until required.

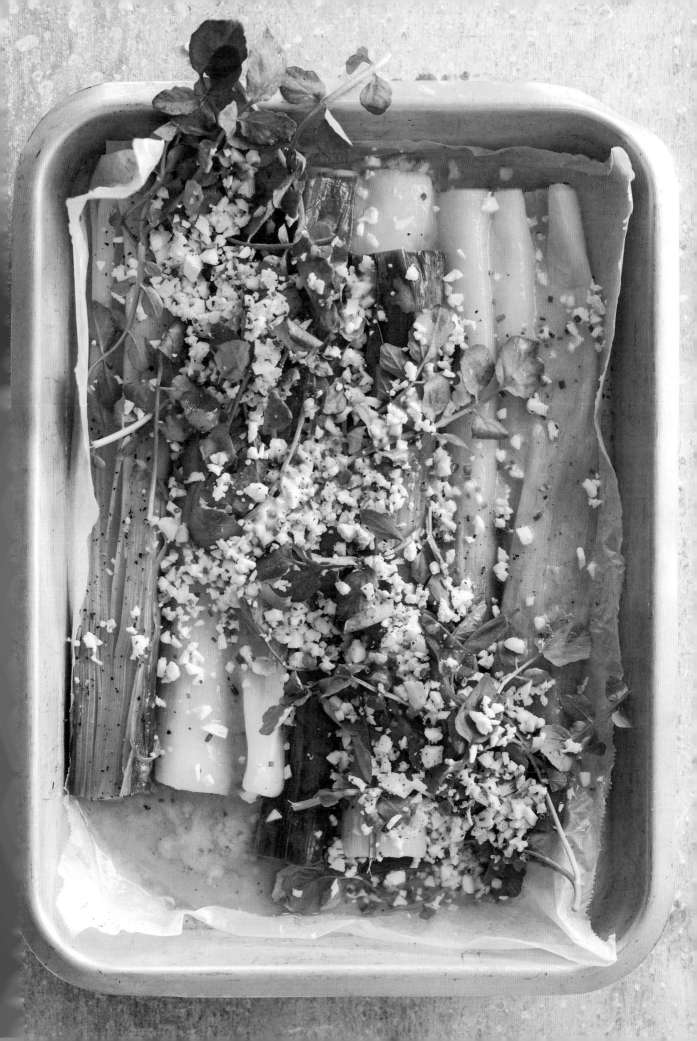

PREPARATION TIME	COOKING TIME	SERVES
30 minutes, plus overnight soaking	35 minutes (including 20 minutes resting)	4

We serve this salad at our cafes every winter, often as a side with eggs. We like using jap pumpkin because once it's roasted, you can eat the skin as well, which means you use up the whole vegetable and do not have to throw anything away; also see our tip at the end of the recipe for using pumpkin seeds.

Lemon myrtle is an indigenous Australian spice that works really well with the richness of the pumpkin. If you can't find it locally, it's definitely worth buying from an online spice supplier, as it is also beautiful in baking. Otherwise, you can just use extra lemon zest.

CRUSTED PUMPKIN & LENTIL SALAD

100 g (3½ oz/½ cup) brown lentils, soaked in water overnight
3–4 flat-leaf (Italian) parsley stems
1 garlic clove, peeled
½ onion, peeled
¼ teaspoon salt
1 handful of picked dill sprigs

FOR THE PUMPKIN
750 g (1 lb 10 oz) jap or kent pumpkin (winter squash)
60 ml (2 fl oz/¼ cup) vegetable oil
zest of ½ lemon
1 cm (½ inch) knob of fresh ginger, grated
1 garlic clove, crushed
½ teaspoon ground lemon myrtle
¼ teaspoon salt

FOR THE CRUST
2 tablespoons pepitas (pumpkin seeds)
1 tablespoon buckwheat
1 tablespoon sesame seeds

BALSAMIC & MUSTARD DRESSING
2 teaspoons apple balsamic vinegar (or 1 teaspoon balsamic vinegar and 1 teaspoon apple cider vinegar)
1 teaspoon dijon mustard
1 teaspoon reserved lentil cooking liquid

Rinse the lentils and wash them well. Place in a large saucepan and cover with water, to a depth of three finger-widths. Add the parsley stems, garlic and onion and bring to the boil over medium heat. Turn the heat down to low and simmer for 15–20 minutes. Turn off the heat, add the salt and let the lentils sit for about 20 minutes. Drain the lentils, reserving 1 teaspoon of the cooking liquid.

Meanwhile, preheat the oven to 180–200°C (350–400°F). Line a baking tray with baking paper. Leaving the skin on the pumpkin, remove the seeds (see tip), then cut the flesh into 3–4 cm (1¼–1½ inch) wedges. In a small bowl, mix together the vegetable oil, lemon zest, ginger, garlic, lemon myrtle and salt. Brush the mixture over both sides of the pumpkin wedges, reserving the remaining oil mixture, and place them on the lined baking tray. Bake for 30–35 minutes, or until golden brown, turning the wedges over after 15 minutes.

To prepare the crust, toast the pepitas, buckwheat and sesame seeds separately in a dry frying pan over medium–low heat until golden brown and fragrant. Chop the pepitas finely and mix with the buckwheat and sesame seeds. Set aside.

To make the dressing, whisk together the vinegar, mustard and some salt and pepper in a small bowl. Slowly whisk in the reserved oil mixture from the pumpkin, and the reserved lentil cooking liquid, until emulsified.

Spread the crust mixture on a large flat plate. When the baked pumpkin wedges are cool enough to handle, lightly press them into the crust mixture, on both sides. Place them on a serving plate.

In a large bowl, mix the drained lentils gently with the dressing and half the dill.

Place the lentils over and between the crusted pumpkin wedges. Garnish with the remaining dill. Serve warm.

TIP: Keep the pumpkin seeds, toss them in a bit of olive oil and salt, spread them on a baking tray lined with baking paper and toast in a 160°C (315°F) oven for 5–8 minutes, or until crisp, and enjoy as a snack. For the crust, try other toasted seeds or nuts, such as chopped almonds or walnuts, or any puffed grains (no roasting needed). Green or even black lentils are beautiful with this recipe too.

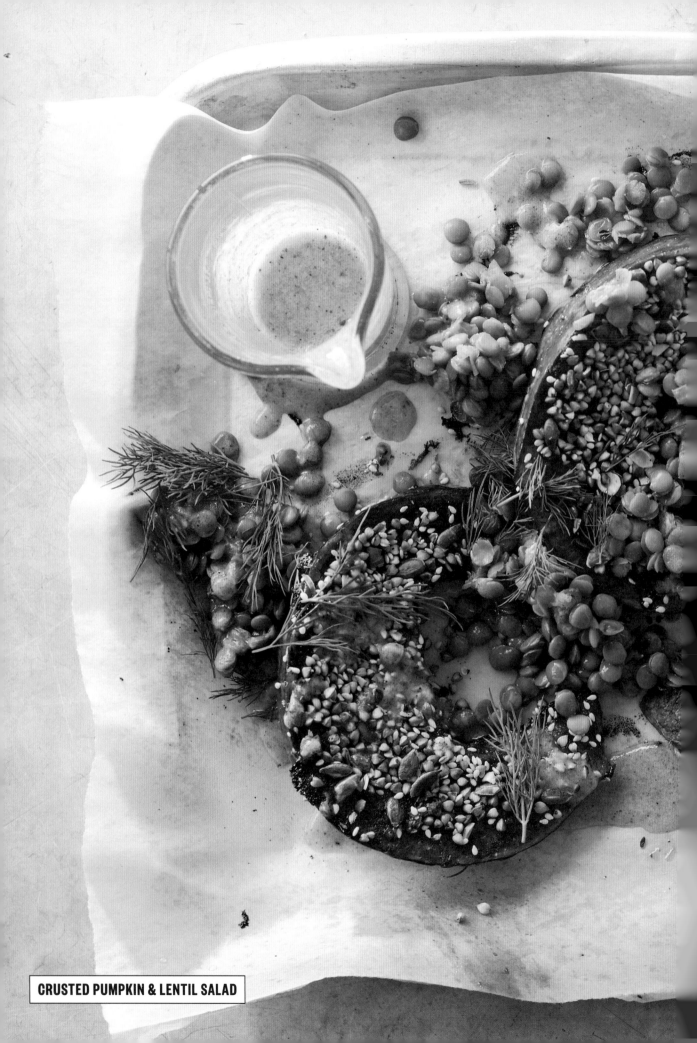

CRUSTED PUMPKIN & LENTIL SALAD

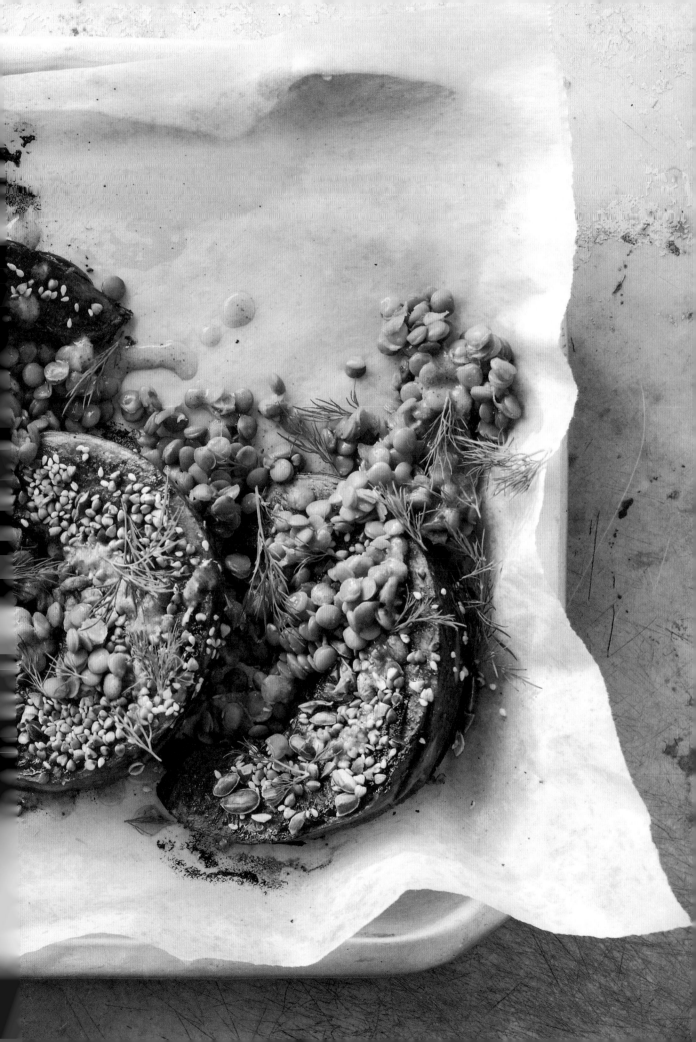

Tangy, rich and spicy, this dish makes a fabulous wintery vegetarian meal. Quinoa is a gluten-free alternative to couscous. Most quinoa comes from South America, but we source ours from a great Tasmanian producer.

Try this dish with parsnips instead of carrots, and any other grains in your pantry.

BRAISED CARROTS WITH QUINOA & TAHINI DRESSING

120 g (4 oz/⅔ cup) quinoa
1½ tablespoons olive oil
600 g (1 lb 5 oz) carrots, peeled and cut into 5−6 cm (2−2½ inch) sticks
1 cinnamon stick
4 cardamom pods, crushed to release their flavour
juice of 2 lemons, and 4 long strips of lemon peel
juice of 2 oranges, and 4 long strips of orange peel
2 garlic cloves, finely crushed
2 thyme sprigs
½ teaspoon ground cumin
¼ teaspoon ground caraway seeds
½ teaspoon ground coriander
⅛ teaspoon ground turmeric
150 ml (5 fl oz) white wine
2 teaspoons honey
1½ tablespoons finely snipped chives
¼ cup picked chervil

TAHINI DRESSING
1 garlic clove, crushed
2 tablespoons tahini
6 tablespoons reserved carrot braising liquid
pinch of cayenne pepper

Soak the quinoa in water for about 15 minutes. Drain and rinse until the water runs clear. Place in a small saucepan, add 150 ml (5 fl oz) water and two pinches of salt and bring to the boil. Reduce the heat and simmer for 10−12 minutes, then turn off the heat, put the lid on and leave to steam for 10−15 minutes.

Meanwhile, heat the olive oil in a heavy-based saucepan over medium−high heat. Add the carrots, cinnamon stick, cardamom pods, and all the citrus peel strips. Season with salt and pepper. Sauté for about 5 minutes, or until the spices are fragrant.

Add the garlic and thyme sprigs and cook, stirring, for another 2−3 minutes. Stir in all the ground spices and fry them off for a few minutes, until fragrant. Add the wine and allow to reduce until it has almost evaporated. Add the lemon and orange juice and reduce for 2 minutes.

Stir in the honey and 150 ml (5 fl oz) water. Cover and simmer for about 20 minutes, or until the carrots are soft. Take the lid off and allow the cooking liquid to reduce for another 2 minutes. Let the carrots cool in the cooking liquid.

Meanwhile, whisk the dressing ingredients in a small bowl until well combined. Season with salt and pepper.

To serve, run a fork through the warm quinoa to fluff up the grains. Spread the quinoa around a serving plate. Arrange the carrots on top and drizzle with a bit of their braising juices. Drizzle the dressing over the salad and garnish with the chives and chervil. Serve warm.

TIP: The braising liquid from the carrots is full of flavour; we use it as the base of the dressing for this dish. Always save your braising liquids when cooking vegetables, to use in dressings, sauces or even in soups.

PREPARATION TIME	COOKING TIME	SERVES
20 minutes, plus overnight soaking	50 minutes, plus 15 minutes soaking	4

Roasting the chickpeas intensifies the flavour of this warm salad — an old favourite, perfect for a cold night. We use our Red Pepper Relish here, made in summer when capsicums are abundant (see page 86), but if you don't have a jar lurking in your pantry, use roasted peppers in oil from your local deli.

POTATO & ROASTED CHICKPEA SALAD WITH RED PEPPER & SHEEP'S FETA

250 g (9 oz/1¼ cups) dried chickpeas, soaked in water overnight

300 g (10½ oz) small to medium-sized waxy (boiling) potatoes, such as Dutch creams, skins scrubbed

1 teaspoon finely chopped Salt-Preserved Citrus Skins (page 187), or preserved lemon rind

2 tablespoons olive oil, plus extra for drizzling over the salad

1 garlic clove, crushed

½ teaspoon smoked paprika

2 tablespoons sherry vinegar (or red wine vinegar if not available)

3 tablespoons Red Pepper Relish (page 86)

2–4 tablespoons chickpea cooking liquid (reserved from above)

2 spring onions (scallions), sliced into thin rings

1 handful of picked flat-leaf (Italian) parsley

125 g (4½ oz) sheep's feta

1–2 tablespoons olive oil

Drain and rinse the chickpeas. Place them in a large saucepan and cover with water, to a depth of three finger-widths. Bring to the boil, skim off any impurities, then reduce the heat and simmer for 30–45 minutes, or until they are tender but still retain their shape. Add a few pinches of salt and leave to sit for about 15 minutes, for the chickpeas to absorb the salt.

Meanwhile, place the potatoes in a saucepan, cover them with cold water, add a few pinches of salt and cook for 20–25 minutes, or until tender. Drain off the water. When cool enough to handle, peel the potatoes, then cut into 1 cm (½ inch) cubes.

Place the potato cubes in a large mixing bowl. Add the citrus skin or preserved lemon rind and season with pepper; you may not need salt, as the citrus element is already very salty.

When the chickpeas are done, heat the olive oil in a large frying pan over high heat. Drain the chickpeas, reserving 2–4 tablespoons of the cooking liquid, and immediately add them to the pan. Season with salt and pepper and stir-fry for 3–4 minutes, or until they start to turn golden brown. Add the garlic and paprika and stir-fry for another 1–2 minutes.

Pour the hot chickpeas over the potato mixture and gently combine. Add the vinegar, red pepper relish and reserved chickpea cooking liquid and mix together gently with a wooden spoon. Let the mixture cool for 5 minutes or so, then fold the spring onion and parsley through.

Place the salad in a bowl or on a platter. Crumble the feta over, finish with a drizzle of olive oil and serve.

TIP: Cook up some extra chickpeas and make some hummus at the same time. The chickpeas need to be soaked overnight before using, but can be cooked a day ahead if this is more convenient.

PREPARATION TIME	COOKING TIME	SERVES
30 minutes	about 40 minutes	4

This rustic recipe is a beautiful combination of winter flavours, and another great example of using the whole vegetable, stem and all. It is also a good way to use up stale sourdough bread.

The roasted cauliflower florets are also delicious with the walnut dip on page 196.

BARBECUED CAULIFLOWER WITH ALMOND & HERBS

Cook the cauliflower in a large saucepan of boiling water for 12–15 minutes, or until the core is just tender. Remove from the water and allow to cool for a few minutes.

Meanwhile, heat the butter and 2 tablespoons of the olive oil in a frying pan over medium heat. Add the breadcrumbs and brown them, stirring constantly, for 3–4 minutes. Stir in the garlic and lemon zest and cook until fragrant. Remove from the heat and place in a bowl to cool.

Heat a barbecue or chargrill pan to medium–high. Place the cooled cauliflower on a plate, season with salt, pepper and the nutmeg, then drizzle with the remaining 1 tablespoon olive oil.

Place the cauliflower on the hot barbecue or chargrill pan, stalk end down. Cook for 5–7 minutes, then turn it onto its other side and cook for another 8–10 minutes, or until evenly browned or charred. Remove from the heat and leave until cool enough to handle.

Toss the parsley, almonds and onion through your toasted bread mixture, mixing well. Check the seasoning.

Break the cauliflower into florets and place on a serving plate. Top with the bread and almond mixture. Drizzle with the lemon juice and a little more olive oil and serve.

½ cauliflower, about 400 g (14 oz)
15 g (½ oz) butter
60 ml (2 fl oz/¼ cup) olive oil, plus extra for drizzling over the salad
50 g (1¾ oz) stale bread, crusts removed, blitzed to coarse breadcrumbs using a food processor
1 garlic clove, crushed
zest and juice of ½ lemon
pinch of freshly grated nutmeg
1 handful of picked flat-leaf (Italian) parsley
2–3 tablespoons toasted almonds (see page 206), coarsely chopped
½ red onion, thinly sliced using a mandoline

PREPARATION TIME	STORAGE	MAKES
20 minutes, plus 20 minutes sterilising	up to 6 months	4 x 300 ml (10½ fl oz) jars

This recipe is based on seasonal vegetables and herbs, pureéd into a concentrated paste and preserved with salt. It can be used as a replacement for stock or stock cubes, by dissolving 1–2 teaspoons in 500 ml (17 fl oz/2 cups) boiling water and adding to stews, soups, risottos or any meals needing a boost of flavour.

The aim here is to use up excess vegetable parts — such as carrot tops, fennel tops, celery leaves, and parsley and coriander stems. A good idea is to save your vegetable scraps in a container in the fridge and make a bouillon at the end of the week. You can use any vegetable that you would normally use when making a stock — just avoid starchy vegies such as potato or pumpkin (winter squash).

The ratio is 1 kg (2 lb 4 oz) vegetables to 250 g (9 oz) salt. Then add a whole bulb of garlic and some preserved lemon or sun-dried tomatoes for extra flavour. You can scale down this basic ratio, making a half or quarter quantity in fewer jars.

VEGIE SCRAP BOUILLON

250 g (9 oz) sea or river salt

1 KG (2 LB 4 OZ) FRESH
    PRODUCE, SUCH AS:
onions (no skin)
leeks (including the thick green
    leafy tops)
shallots (no skin)
spring onions (scallions)
garlic (no skin)
carrots and green leafy tops
fennel and fronds
celery and leaves
celeriac (including the skin
    peelings, if washed well)
parsley leaves, stems and
    well-washed roots
coriander (cilantro) leaves,
    stems and well-washed roots
thyme sprigs
sun-dried tomatoes
preserved lemons (including the
    flesh), or Salt-Preserved Citrus
    Skins from page 187

Sterilise your jars and lids (see page 212). Leave to cool to room temperature.

Meanwhile, using a large sharp knife, chop all your fresh produce into 2–3 cm (¾–1½ inch) chunks.

In batches if necessary, add the ingredients to a food processor with the salt. Process into a thick paste.

Pack the paste into the jars, making sure the paste doesn't touch the inside of the lids, if you are using metal ones, as the salt can cause them to rust.

Remove any air bubbles by gently tapping each jar on the work surface and sliding a clean butter knife or chopstick around the inside to release any hidden air pockets. Wipe the rims of the jars with paper towel or a clean damp cloth and seal.

Your bouillon will keep in a cool, dark place for up to 6 months. Once opened, refrigerate and use within 1 year.

TIP: You could also make a few jars of a spicy Asian-flavoured paste to use in noodle soups, stir-fries, and marinades for chicken and fish. Follow the same steps as above, but halve the recipe to make only two 300 ml (10½ fl oz) jars, using 125 g (4½ oz) salt and about 500 g (1 lb 2 oz) fresh produce, such as chillies; peeled garlic, onion and/or shallots; ginger and/or galangal (including the peel); lemongrass (including the long leaves); fennel and/or carrot (including the green tops).

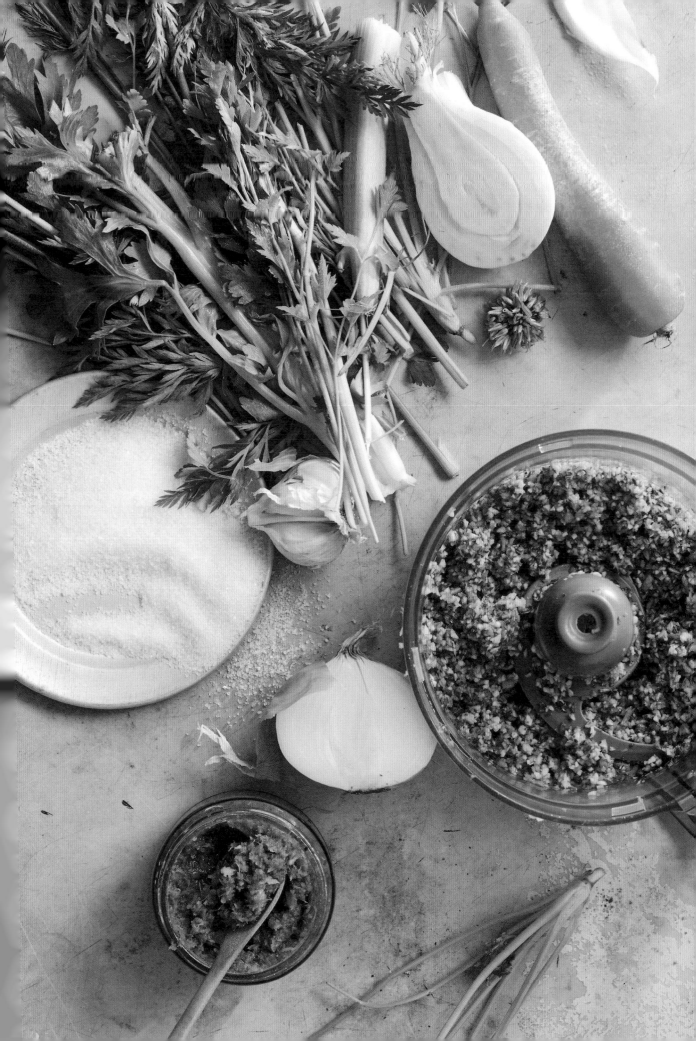

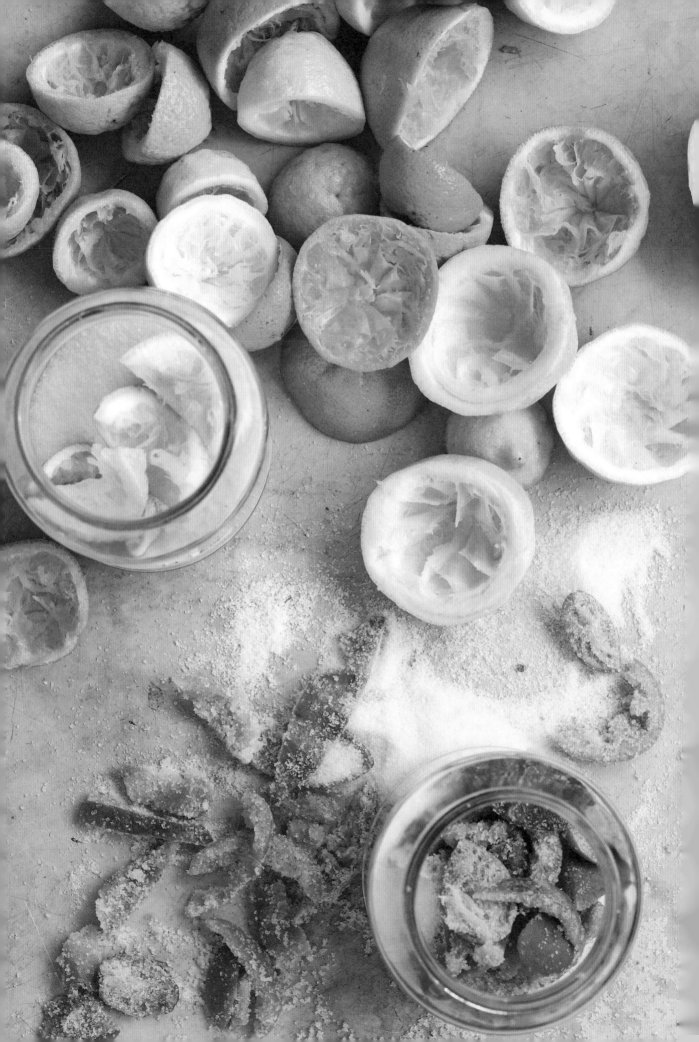

PREPARATION TIME	PRESERVING TIME	STORAGE	MAKES
10 minutes	6 weeks	up to 2 years	1 x 1–2 litre (35–70 fl oz/4–8 cup) jar

Everyone is always asking us how to use citrus skins once the fruit has been juiced. This recipe isn't as fancy as preserved lemons, but is a great way to reduce kitchen waste and at the same time produce a delicious kitchen staple. It is similar to preserving lemons, except you're using 100% salt to preserve the citrus skins, and no citrus juice. And you can combine all different kinds of citrus skins in the one jar — there is no need to preserve them in separate jars.

When a recipe calls for preserved lemons or citrus peel, you can fish a bit of your salt-preserved citrus skin out of the jar, rinse it or soak it for 30 minutes, then thinly slice it to use in stews, soups, tagines, marinades and dressings.

SALT-PRESERVED CITRUS SKINS

Give your jar and lid a good wash and make sure they are completely dry inside. (If you'd prefer to sterilise them, follow the instructions on page 212.)

Put a layer of cooking salt in the bottom of the jar, about 3 cm (1¼ inches) deep. Each time you squeeze a lemon, orange or lime, flatten the peel with the palm of your hand and press it into the salt, then cover the skins with more salt. You can cut the citrus peel into strips to speed up the preserving process — just make sure all the skins are buried under the salt.

As time passes, the salt and citrus peel will compress down and you'll be able to keep adding more to the jar. The peel will be ready to use after about 6 weeks.

If you're using a jar with a metal lid, just be mindful that the salt doesn't reach the top of the jar and corrode the metal.

As the citrus peels release their juices, moisture will start to build up at the bottom of the jar — don't worry about this, as there is so much salt in the jar that no bacteria will be able to grow.

The jar will happily sit on the benchtop indefinitely, but during a heatwave we like to store it in the fridge.

lots of pure salt or cooking salt
citrus skins, such as lemon, lime, mandarin or orange

PREPARATION TIME	COOKING TIME	STORAGE	MAKES
30 minutes, plus 20 minutes sterilising, plus 10 minutes heat-processing	1 hour	up to 2 years	4–5 x 300 ml (10½ fl oz) jars

When we serve this chutney in our cooking class lunches, our students try to lick the bowl! Here is the recipe, for everyone who has ever asked for it. This chutney is very versatile — we serve it with eggs and on wraps, and it's great as a table condiment. You'll definitely be asked to share the recipe.

PUMPKIN & SESAME CHUTNEY

2 kg (4 lb 8 oz) sweet pumpkin (winter squash), such as jap or kent; all up you'll need 1.5 kg (3 lb 5 oz) pumpkin flesh for this recipe
125 ml (4 fl oz/½ cup) vegetable oil
2 teaspoons salt
500 g (1 lb 2 oz) onions
40 g (1½ oz) knob of fresh ginger
2 garlic cloves
2 teaspoons black mustard seeds
1 teaspoon ground cumin
pinch of cayenne pepper
1 tablespoon toasted sesame seeds (see page 206)
110 g (3¾ oz/½ cup) white sugar
50 g (1¾ oz/¼ cup) brown sugar
500 ml (17 fl oz/2 cups) apple cider vinegar

Preheat the oven to 180°C (350°F). Prepare the pumpkin by removing the skin, core and seeds. Cut the flesh into 5 cm (2 inch) chunks, place on a baking tray with 60 ml (2 fl oz/¼ cup) of the oil and ½ teaspoon of the salt. Bake for 40 minutes, or until soft and caramelised.

While the pumpkin is roasting, peel and thinly slice the onions. Peel and crush the garlic, and wash and grate the ginger.

Warm the remaining oil in a large, shallow and wide non-reactive saucepan over medium heat and sauté the onion, stirring often, for about 8 minutes, or until soft and translucent. Add the garlic and ginger. Stir in the mustard seeds, cumin, cayenne pepper and sesame seeds and cook for a few minutes.

Mix the roasted pumpkin through; it will fall apart as you do this. Add all the sugar, the vinegar and remaining salt. Stir to combine, then reduce the heat and cook for 15–20 minutes, stirring often. Because the pumpkin is already cooked, this chutney won't take too long to reach the right consistency. It should be thick, with no puddles of vinegar on the surface — you'll be able to run your wooden spoon through and see the bottom of the pan for a few seconds. If it's too dry, you can loosen it up by stirring in a little more vinegar or water.

Meanwhile, sterilise your jars and lids (see page 212).

Carefully fill the hot jars with the hot relish. Remove any air bubbles by gently tapping each jar on the work surface and sliding a clean butter knife or chopstick around the inside to release any hidden air pockets. Wipe the rims of the jars with paper towel or a clean damp cloth and seal immediately.

Heat-process the jars (see page 211) for 10 minutes. Leave to cool on the benchtop, then store in a cool, dark place for up to 2 years. Try to let the chutney sit for at least 1 month before eating. Once opened, store in the fridge and use within 6 months.

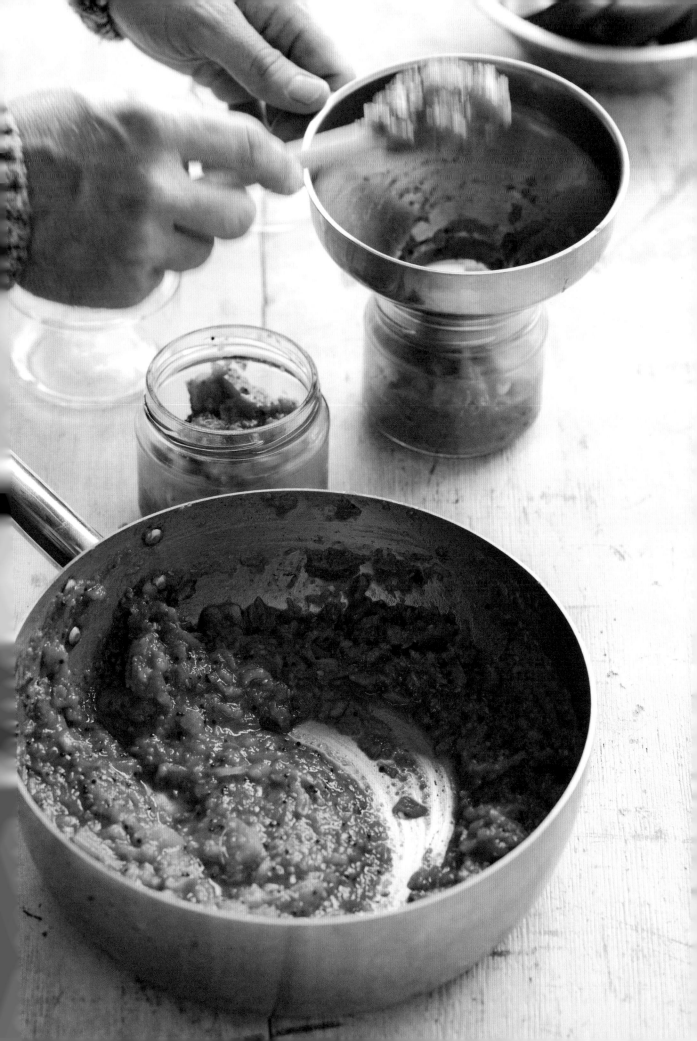

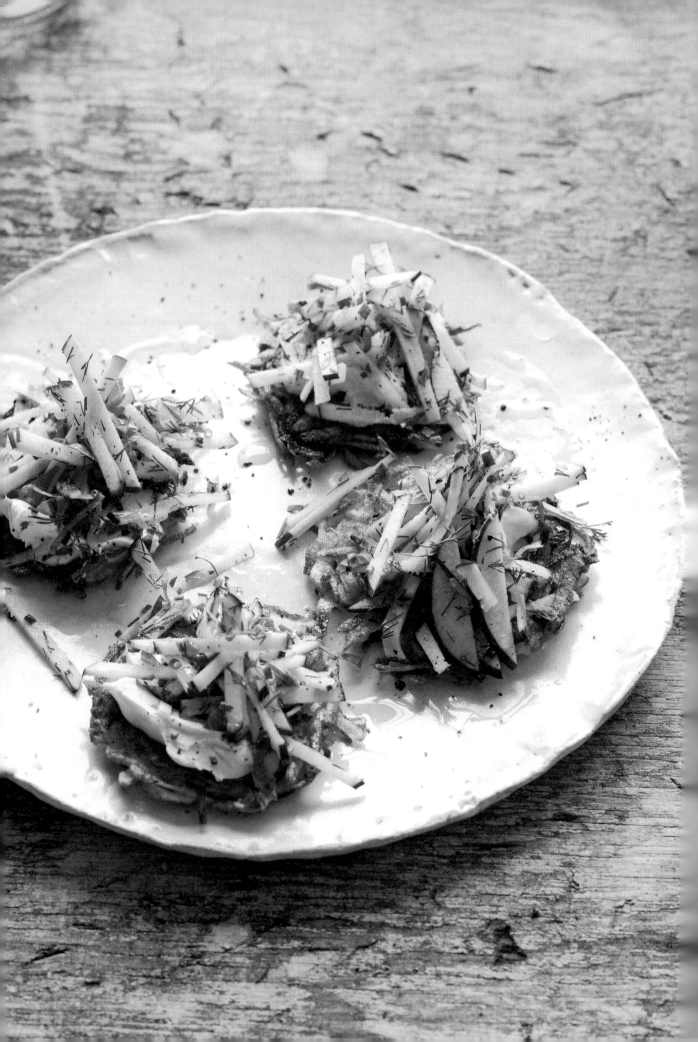

PREPARATION TIME	COOKING TIME	SERVES
30 minutes	about 20 minutes	4

This dish is delicious. Everyone loves it and it's so pretty on a platter. We even eat it for breakfast! You can serve the radish and apple salad with other meals too bulking it out with some shaved cabbage.

RADISH & APPLE SALAD ON POTATO RÖSTI

Preheat the oven to about 75°C (170°F).

To make the rösti, peel the potatoes, then coarsely grate them into a clean tea towel. Fold the tea towel together and squeeze out as much moisture as possible. Season the grated potatoes with the nutmeg and freshly ground pepper, then divide into eight equal portions.

Place a frying pan, large enough to cook four rösti at a time, over medium heat. Add about 2 tablespoons clarified butter and 2 tablespoons vegetable oil. Place four rösti into the pan, pressing them down with the back of a spoon and giving them a round shape. Fry the rösti for 4–5 minutes on each side, or until golden brown and crisp on the outside, and tender all the way through, adding more butter or vegetable oil if needed.

Drain on paper towel and season with salt, then place on a wire rack and keep them warm in the oven until serving. Finish cooking the remaining four rösti in the same way, keeping them warm in the oven until serving.

Meanwhile, using a mandoline, thinly slice the apples and radishes, then cut them into matchsticks. Place in a large mixing bowl, add the chopped herbs and gently mix together. Season with salt and pepper, add the vinegar and olive oil and gently mix again.

Place the warm röstis on a platter or individual serving plates. Arrange the salad on top and finish with a dollop of crème fraiche, or spread the crème fraiche over the rösti and top with the salad. Serve immediately.

2 small apples
4 large radishes
2 tablespoons finely chopped dill
2 tablespoons finely snipped chives
2 tablespoons coarsely chopped
    flat-leaf (Italian) parsley
1 tablespoon sherry vinegar
2 tablespoons olive oil
4 tablespoons crème fraiche or
    sour cream

FOR THE RÖSTI
800 g–1 kg (1 lb 12 oz–2 lb 4 oz)
    potatoes
2 pinches of freshly grated
    nutmeg
clarified butter or ghee,
    for pan-frying
vegetable oil, for pan-frying

TIP: Leftover herbs will stay fresh for at least a week if you wrap them in a slightly damp paper towel and keep them in a sealed plastic bag in the crisper. This also works for lettuce and kale. You could also save your herb stems for a batch of Vegie Scrap Bouillon on page 184, or the Cornersmith Chimichurri on page 37. Save your radish tops for the Kitchen Scrap Sauerkraut on page 192.

PREPARATION TIME	FERMENTING TIME	STORAGE	MAKES
40 minutes, plus 20 minutes sterilising	2 days to 2 weeks	up to 6 months	2 x 500 ml (17 fl oz/2 cup) jars

This sauerkraut recipe comes from Cornersmith's head fermenter and teacher, Jaimee Edwards. It's a very flexible one in which you can use up vegetable stems and leaves, or those bits lurking in the back of the fridge. Altogether you'll need 2 kg (4 lb 8 oz) of produce, including 500 g (1 lb 2 oz) fruit and vegie 'scraps'.

Flavour the sauerkraut with whole spices or herbs to match your vegetable combinations. Caraway seeds are a classic with cabbage, apple and onion; black peppercorns go well with warrigal greens, fennel and beetroot leaves; and kale and dill are really delicious together.

KITCHEN SCRAP SAUERKRAUT

1.5 kg (3 lb 5 oz) white cabbage
500 g (1 lb 2 oz) assorted leftover fruit and vegetable bits, such as onions, apples, pears, chokos (chayotes), kohlrabi, silverbeet (Swiss chard) leaves, and the chopped stems and leaves from parsley, dill, beetroot (beet), fennel, kale, celery and warrigal greens

1 tablespoon salt
1 tablespoon whole spices of your choice, such as juniper berries, caraway seeds, bay leaves and black or white peppercorns

Sterilise your jars and lids (see page 212). Leave to cool to room temperature.

Meanwhile, cut the cabbage into manageable pieces, and shred any smaller portions of cabbage into thin strips. Place in a non-reactive bowl large enough to hold all your produce.

If you are using apples or pears, cut them into thin strips and set aside. Cut your other vegetables and greens to about the same size as your cabbage, then add them to the bowl.

Sprinkle the salt on the cabbage mixture and mix thoroughly with your hands. Using a pestle, or a rolling pin without a handle – or even the top side of a meat mallet – pound your produce until a lot of the water is released. You should be able to grab a fist full of the mixture, give it a squeeze, and see brine running freely. At this stage your sauerkraut is ready to jar up. If you are using apples or pears, mix them through now.

Add the sauerkraut to your jars and pack down very tightly, to about 2 cm (¾ inch) from the rim of the jars, allowing about 1 cm (½ inch) of the brine from your produce to cover the top of the mixture. This is very important to prevent spoilage.

Seal your jars and place out of direct sunlight. In temperate weather, leave to ferment for at least 4 days; in summer, it is advisable to check on your sauerkraut after 2 days, as fermentation will happen much more quickly.

Open your jar every few days to 'burp' your ferment – this will release the built-up carbon dioxide, and prevent brine spilling out of the jar. Just be sure to press down your sauerkraut afterwards, so that the brine is covering the top by at least 1 cm (½ inch).

You may leave your sauerkraut to ferment for 2 weeks, checking every few days to see and taste how it is developing.

Once you are happy with your sauerkraut, refrigerate for up to 6 months.

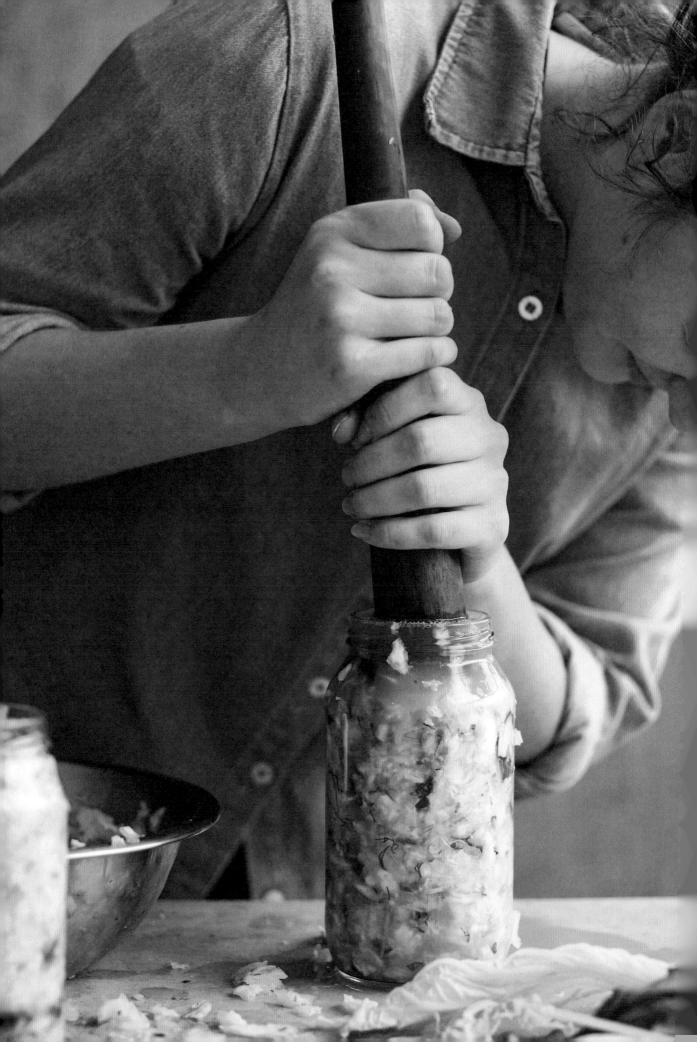

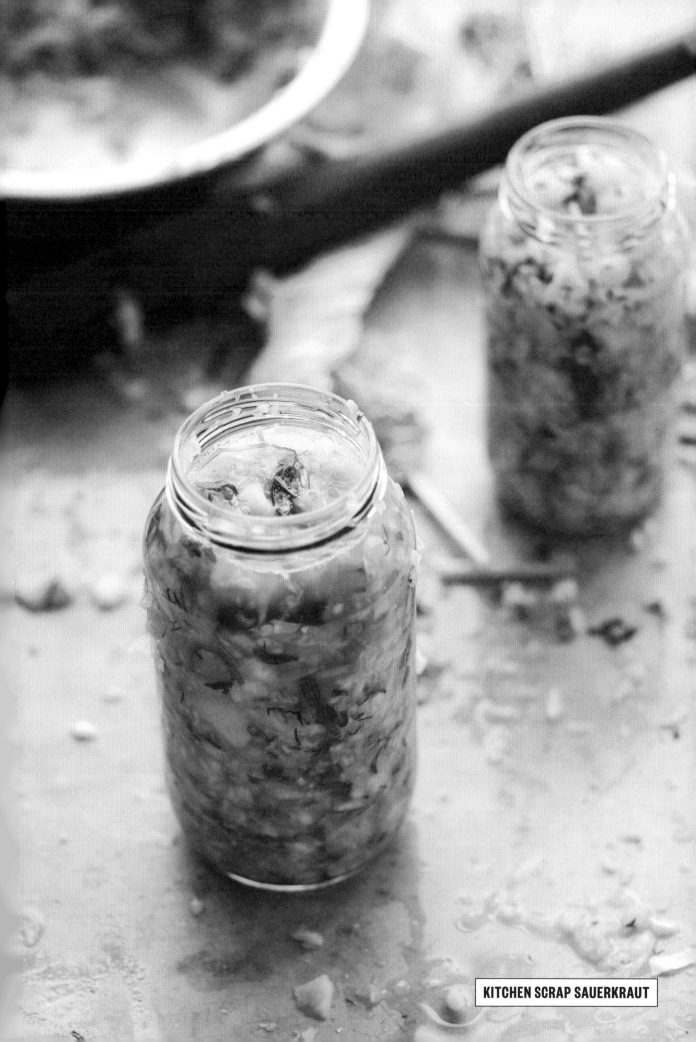

KITCHEN SCRAP SAUERKRAUT

PREPARATION TIME	COOKING TIME	SERVES
25 minutes	about 10 minutes	4

When it's walnut season, make the most of it with this delicious dip. In the Middle East, this kind of dip is often served with flat bread or alongside grilled meats. We serve it with raw winter vegetables such as carrots, fennel, radish and celery, but it is also lovely spread over crusty sourdough, topped with the Bitter Winter Leaves Salad on page 169. The dip gets better on the second or third day, and will last in an airtight container in the fridge for up to 5 days.

RAW VEGETABLES WITH WALNUT & PAPRIKA DIP

1 tablespoon olive oil,
    for pan-frying
1 brown onion, finely diced
3 garlic cloves, finely crushed
¼ teaspoon sweet paprika
120 g (4 oz) stale bread
150 g (5½ oz/1¼ cups) walnuts
    (see tip)
zest and juice of 1 lemon
250 ml (9 fl oz/1 cup) olive oil

TO SERVE
sweet paprika, for sprinkling
4 celery stalks, cut into 6 cm
    (2½ inch) lengths
1 large carrot, cut into long
    wedges or sticks
1 Lebanese (short) cucumber,
    cut into long wedges or sticks
½ fennel bulb, cut into long
    wedges or sticks

Heat the 1 tablespoon of olive oil in a frying pan over medium heat. Add the onion, garlic and paprika and sweat over low heat for about 10 minutes, or until soft, stirring now and then. Set aside.

Meanwhile, cut the crust off the bread, cut the bread into small chunks and soak in 150 ml (5 fl oz) water.

In a food processor, pulse the walnuts into fine crumbs. Add the sautéed onion mixture and blend into a pureé. Add the lemon zest, lemon juice and bread (don't worry about squeezing out the liquid), and pulse again. With the food processor running, add the 250 ml (9 fl oz/ 1 cup) olive oil in a very fine stream (as though you are making a mayonnaise). Add a little more water if the mixture is too thick. Season to taste with salt and pepper.

Transfer to a serving bowl, sprinkle with paprika and serve with the cut vegetables arranged around.

TIP: Lightly toasting the walnuts will intensify the flavour of the dip; just be sure to let them cool completely before using. You can also try this recipe with raw or lightly toasted almonds.

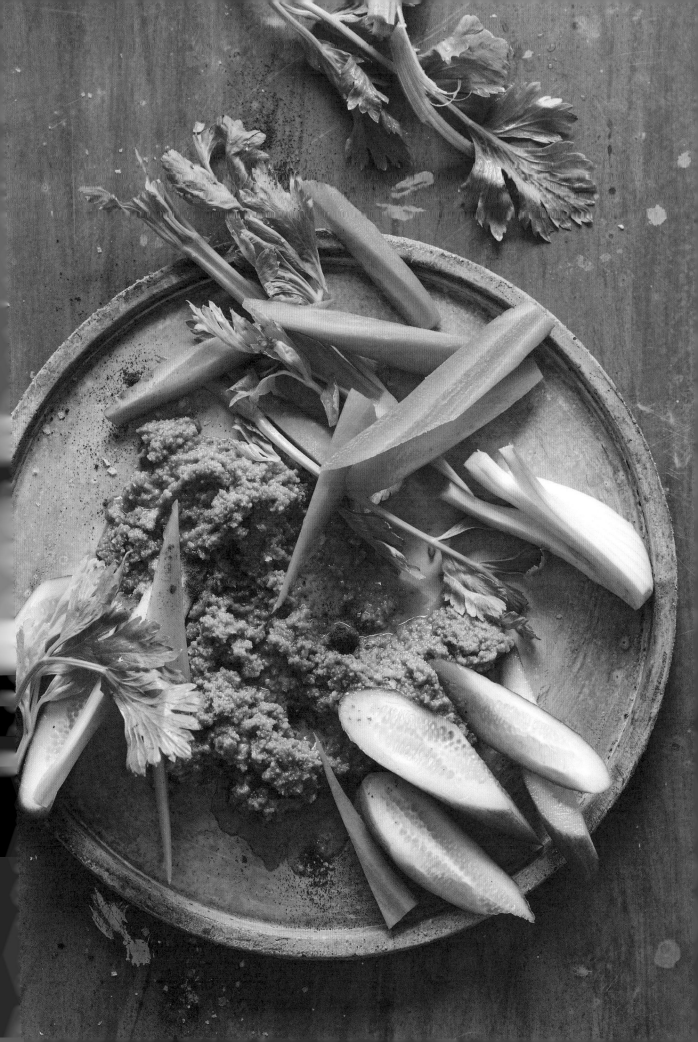

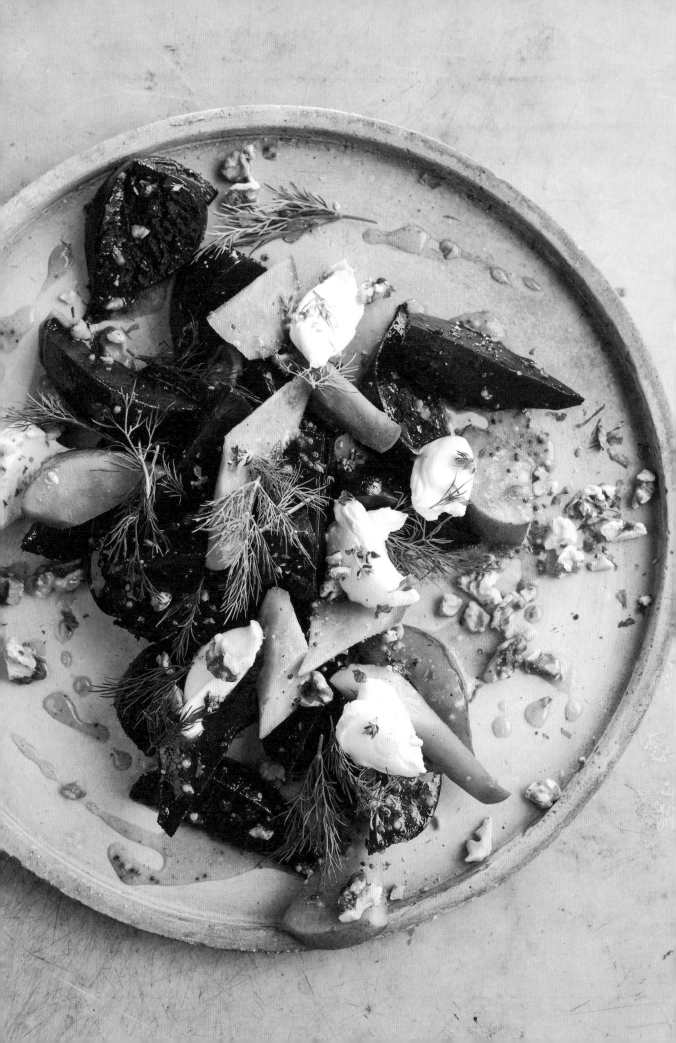

PREPARATION TIME	COOKING TIME	SERVES
20 minutes, plus 5 minutes marinating	1 hour, plus 20 minutes resting	4

This salad is a classic combination of all the best winter produce, with sweet pickled pears adding a Cornersmith spin. If you don't have any Pickled Pears from page 200 on hand, you could use fresh pear, or the roasted pears from the salad on page 106, or any other pickled fruits.

Try this salad as well with feta or goat's cheese instead of labneh, and toasted hazelnuts instead of walnuts.

BAKED BEETROOT WITH SWEET PICKLED PEARS, TOASTED WALNUTS & LABNEH

Preheat the oven to 180°C (350°F).

Lay a piece of baking paper on a large piece of foil. Sprinkle the salt onto the baking paper. Remove the stems from the beetroot, then score the top of each beetroot in a cross shape, using a small sharp knife. Sit the beets, scored end up, on the salt. Add the lemon thyme sprigs, lemon peel strips and garlic cloves. Sprinkle with pepper and tie up the foil, into a parcel.

Place the foil parcel on a baking tray and bake for 1 hour, or until the beetroot is soft. Remove from the oven and leave to cool in the parcel for 15–20 minutes.

To make the dressing, mix the pickling liquid and mustards together in a screw-top jar. Add the olive oil, season with salt and pepper, put the lid on and shake well until the dressing has emulsified.

When the beetroot are cool enough to handle, open the foil parcel and gently peel them. Cut into bite-sized wedges and place in a mixing bowl. Pour half the dressing over them and leave to marinate for about 5 minutes.

Place the beetroot wedges in a serving bowl or on a plate. Arrange the pear and dollops of labneh on top. Sprinkle with the lemon thyme leaves, dill and walnuts. Drizzle the remaining dressing over the salad and serve.

TIP: Pickling liquids and fermenting juices make the best salad dressings. Once you've eaten all your pickles, don't throw away the brines! Just whisk in a little olive oil and mustard.

3 tablespoons coarse salt
4 medium-sized beetroot (beets), washed well
3 lemon thyme sprigs, plus 1 teaspoon picked lemon thyme leaves
3 strips of lemon peel
2 garlic cloves, smashed with the back of a knife
4 Sweet Pickled Pear Quarters (page 200), each quarter cut in half
120 g (4 oz) labneh
½ cup picked dill
40 g (1½ oz/⅓ cup) toasted walnuts (see page 206), roughly chopped

PICKLED PEAR & MUSTARD DRESSING
1 tablespoon pear pickling liquid (from above)
½ teaspoon dijon mustard
½ teaspoon wholegrain mustard
2 tablespoons olive oil

PREPARATION TIME	COOKING TIME	STORAGE	MAKES
30 minutes, plus 20 minutes sterilising, plus 15 minutes heat-processing (optional)	10 minutes	6 months, or up to 2–3 years if heat-processed	3–4 x 500 ml (17 fl oz/2 cup) jars

Alex teaches this pickled pear recipe in her Winter Preserving class and they're a huge hit! Rich and sweet, they are amazing with cheeses, or tossed through salads — Sabine uses them in her baked beetroot salad recipe on page 199. We like to use firm brown-skinned pears such as bosc, but any pears are okay as long as they are very firm. Leaving the skin on helps the pickles hold their shape.

These pickles are lovely after a month, but if you can hold out until December, they are delicious with Christmas ham and also make great Christmas gifts.

Once you've had a chance to enjoy them, don't throw the syrupy brine away — it's amazing in a cocktail or as the base in a salad dressing.

SWEET PICKLED PEARS

500 ml (17 fl oz/2 cups) apple
   cider vinegar
250 ml (9 fl oz/1 cup) water
300 g (10½ oz/1½ cups) brown
   sugar
8 cloves
16 black peppercorns
12 allspice berries
4 bay leaves
1 kg (2 lb 4 oz) firm pears, washed

Sterilise your jars and lids (see page 212).

Meanwhile, make your pickling brine by combining the vinegar, water, sugar and spices in a non-reactive, medium-sized saucepan over low heat. Stir to dissolve the sugar, then bring to simmering point.

Cut the pears into halves or quarters and pack firmly into the jars, leaving 1 cm (½ inch) space at the top.

Bring your brine back up to the boil. Pour the hot brine over the pears, evenly distributing the spices among the jars, and ensuring the pears are completely submerged.

Remove any air bubbles by gently tapping each jar on the work surface and sliding a clean butter knife or chopstick around the inside to release any hidden air pockets. Wipe the rims of the jars with paper towel or a clean damp cloth and seal immediately.

Leave to cool on the benchtop, then store in a cool, dark place for up to 6 months. The pears will be ready to eat after 4 weeks. To extend the shelf life to 2–3 years, heat-process the jars (see page 211) for 15 minutes.

Once opened, store in the fridge and use within 6 months.

TIP: If your pears are really hard you can soften them in the simmering vinegar brine for 10 minutes. You can also make this recipe with peeled and quartered quinces — simmer them until lightly pink and starting to soften, then pickle as above.

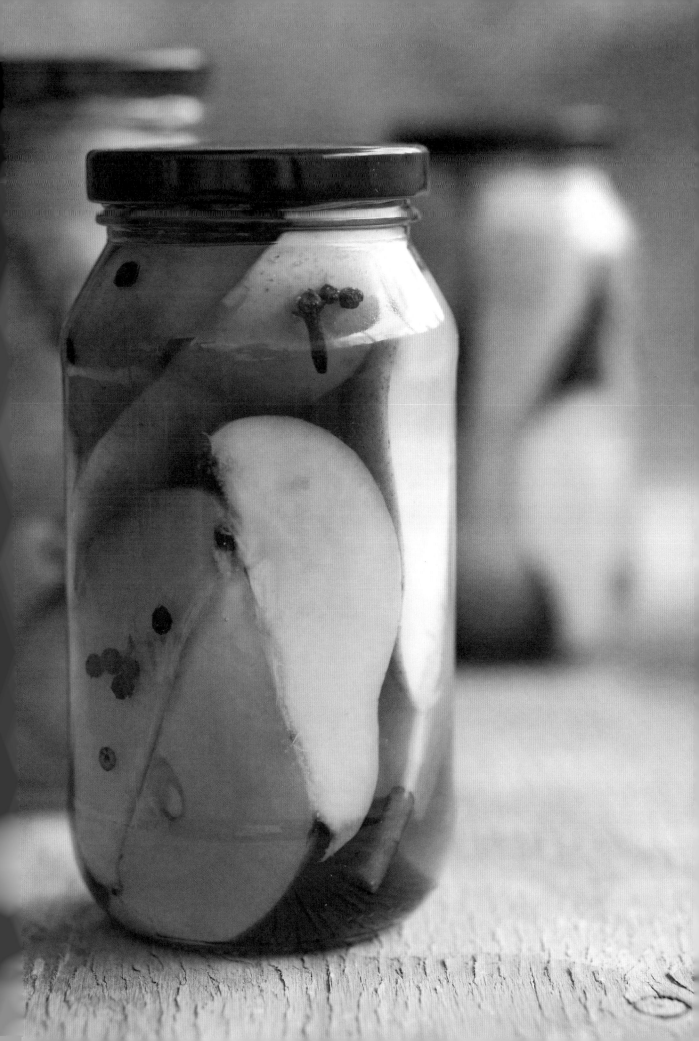

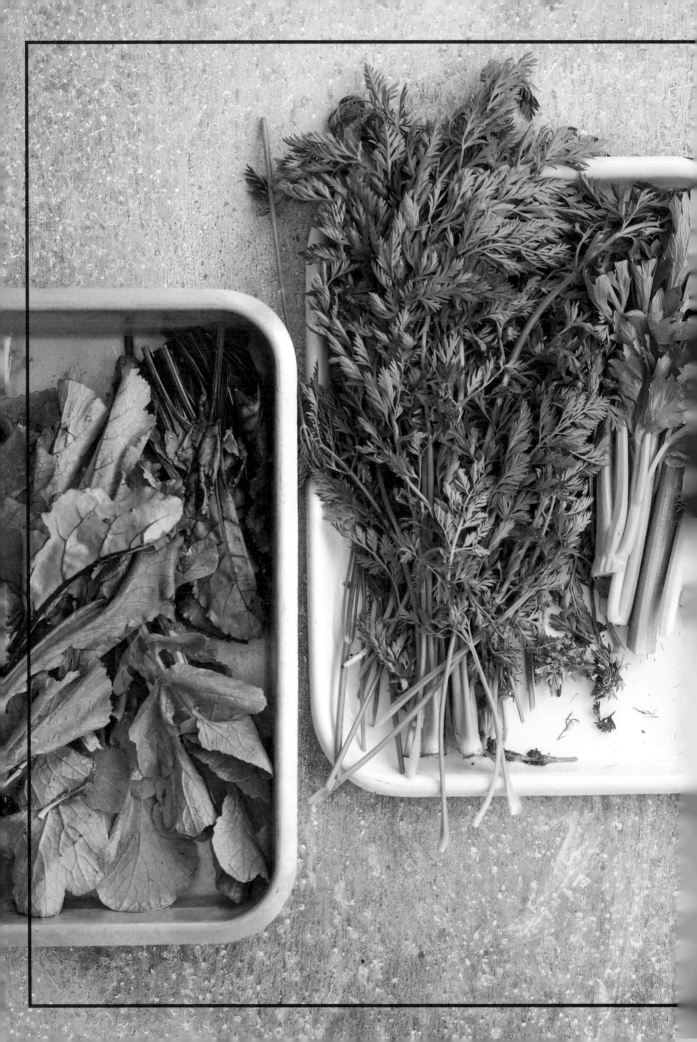

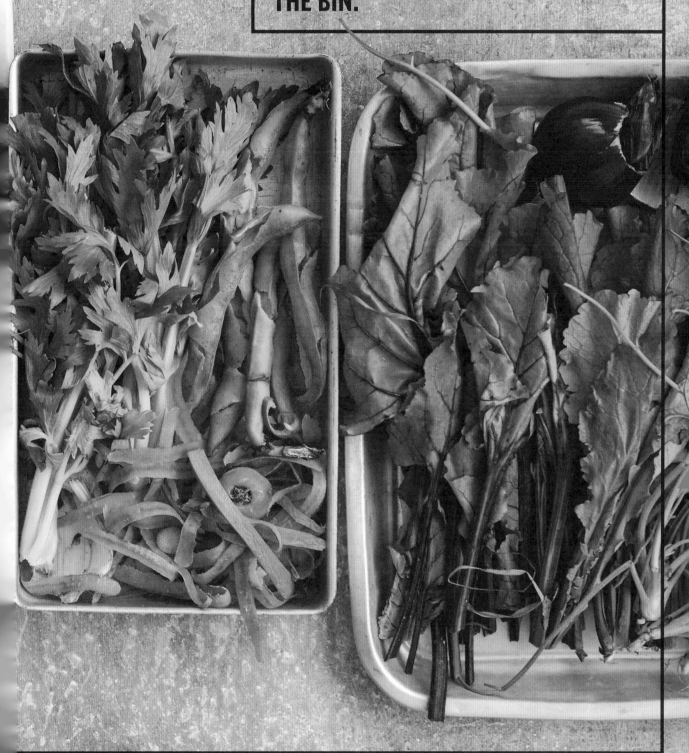

WE NEED TO RETHINK OUR APPROACH TO KITCHEN FOOD WASTE. IT IS TIME TO EXPLORE PRESERVING AND PICKLING, AND TO COME UP WITH WAYS TO EXTRACT MAXIMUM FLAVOUR FROM THE PARTS OF THE INGREDIENT THAT WOULD GENERALLY END UP IN THE BIN.

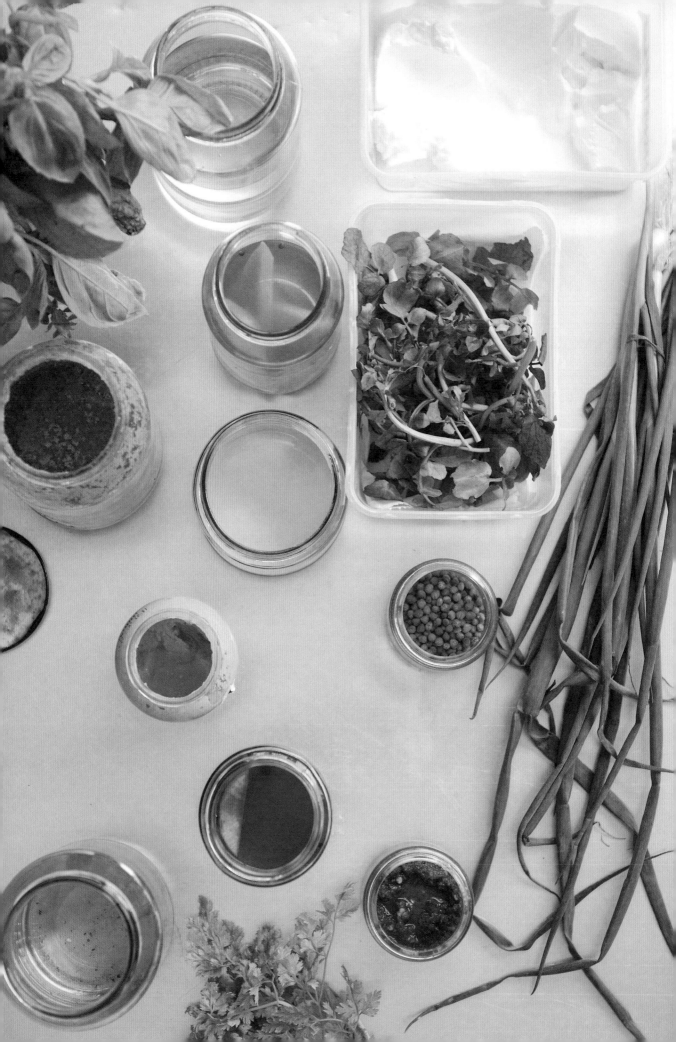

SALAD DRESSING GUIDE

At Cornersmith we focus a lot on salad dressings, finding ways to use up 'by-products' that would normally be thrown out, such as herb stems and leftover pickling and fermenting brines.

Dressings are a light and easy alternative to more involved sauces. They can be as simple and quick to prepare as splashing together a bit of lemon juice, olive oil and a pinch of salt and pepper to dress a salad for a summer picnic, or more complex in flavour, becoming the highlight of a 'showstopper' salad.

Basically you want to find a balance between acidity, saltiness, sweetness and richness in a dressing, tailoring it of course to the dish you are pairing it with.

Here is our base recipe for dressings:

1 part acidity — vinegar or citrus juice, or leftover
    pickling or fermenting brines
2–3 parts oil/fat — any mixture of good-quality
    vegetable, olive or nut oils, or even nut 'butters'
    such as tahini or almond butter
a pinch of seasoning — salt, pepper and any spices
    you'd like to experiment with
a dash of sweetening — a pinch of sugar, a drizzle of
    honey, or any leftover jam or citrus marmalade

Be daring and experiment with using up 'leftover' items in your dressings, such as pickling liquids, fermenting liquids, cheesemaking 'by-products' such as whey, or even yoghurt, buttermilk or kefir.

Using a **pickling or fermenting brine** in a dressing means you probably won't need any vinegar or acidic ingredient, or just a very minimal amount; you will also find that pickling brines are already slightly sweet and have salt and spices added, so be careful not to 'over-season' the dressing, adjusting the seasoning as you go.

When using **dairy products**, you may want to lower your vinegar or acidic component, as they have their own acidity. Also, as dairy products contain fat, you can reduce your oil content as well.

For the **oily/fatty elements** in your dressing, we suggest mixtures of good-quality vegetable oils such as sunflower or grapeseed, and olive or nut oils. Many olive oils or nut oils can be very strong and overpowering in flavour, so bear this in mind, especially if you are also using a pickling or fermenting brine in your dressing, as these are already full of flavour.

If you'd like to play around with **nut butters**, such as tahini, or almond or cashew butter, thin them down with water and a dash of acidity, and reduce the oil content, so the dressing doesn't get too rich.

To add richness, you can also fold a bit of **mayonnaise** into your dressing, which works really well for more rustic dishes such as a potato salad, or as a cold dressing for a piece of grilled meat or fish. As well as being a fantastic cold dressing, a mayonnaise is another great way to use up egg yolks left over from another dish (see page 85). Just be aware that the life span of a mayonnaise is quite short, a maximum of 3 days, as you are using raw egg.

As a **sweetening element**, if needed, you can mix in a little sugar, honey or any leftover marmalade, or use the residual sweetness from a pickling brine.

If you have any **leftover herbs or herb stems** in your fridge, you can easily use these in a herb-based dressing, such as Chimichurri (see page 37), which you can use either as a heavier dressing, or you can fold a small amount into another dressing to add a herbal kick. Of course you can always simply mix some freshly chopped herbs into a dressing, but make sure you do this just before serving the salad, as chopped herbs change flavour very quickly and can't be stored too long.

Be a little adventurous and don't be afraid to try out new things. Any **toasted seeds or nuts** (see right) in your pantry can be used to dress up a simple leaf salad, as can bits of stale bread that you've toasted into **croutons**. And don't forget **sprouted pulses, seeds and grains** (see page 130), to add texture, colour, flavour and an extra burst of nutrition to your salads.

Airtight glass jars are perfect for making dressings in, as well as storing them in the fridge. You can even use jars containing some leftover pickling or fermenting brine as a dressing vessel, then add your new ingredients and then store your dressing in the same jar. Oil-based dressings will generally keep in the fridge for up to a week, or several days if you are using a dairy component.

For convenience, you can make a larger amount of dressing and keep it handy in the fridge for later use; just shake the jar when you take it out of the fridge, and check the seasoning. Dressings containing olive oil may solidify a little on chilling; simply bring them back to room temperature and shake the jar well to emulsify the oil again.

TOASTING SEEDS AND NUTS

Adding toasted seeds or nuts is a very simple and delicious way to turn a straightforward salad into something more interesting. You can of course use raw seeds or nuts, but toasting them enhances their nuttiness and flavour, and is very quick to do.

Preheat your oven to 150°C (300°F). (A lower temperature seems to develop the flavour better, but if you are in a hurry you could bump the oven up to 170°C/325°F.)

Spread your chosen seeds or nuts on a baking tray and toast them in the oven until they turn golden brown and crunchy, and have developed a very nutty flavour.

Put a timer on and move the seeds or nuts around the tray at 2–3 minute intervals, to ensure they toast evenly, and at the same rate.

Small seeds such as **sesame or poppy seeds** might only need just 4–5 minutes at 150°C (300°F); **sunflower seeds, pepitas (pumpkin seeds)** and **buckwheat** 5–7 minutes; and larger nuts such as **almonds, hazelnuts, walnuts** and **pecans** 7–12 minutes.

Leave to cool, then store in an airtight jar in the pantry. They will stay fresh for about a week but try them and if they're a little stale you can give them another 3–5 minutes in the oven.

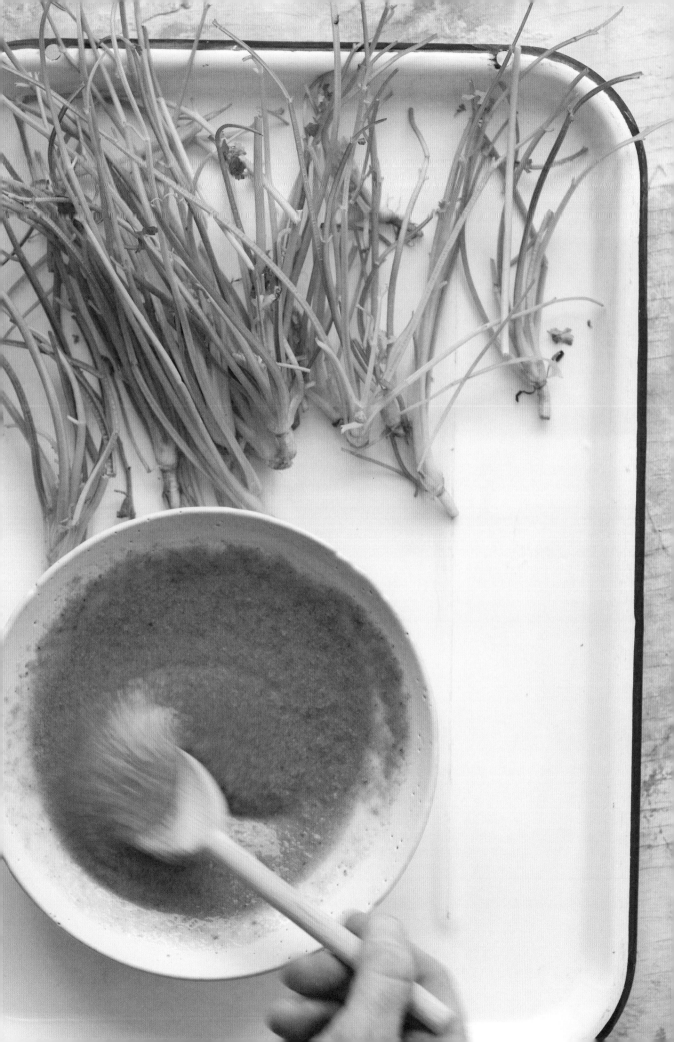

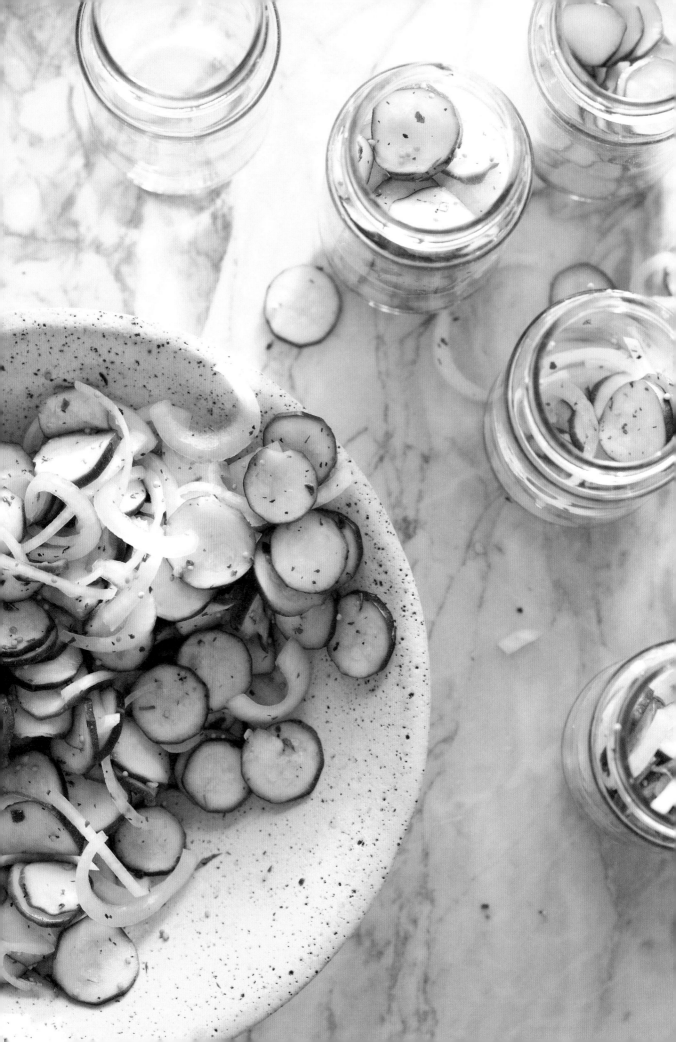

PICKLING GUIDE

Alex's love for pickling started the Cornersmith adventure, and it has become our signature. You'll never get sick of having a pantry full of home-made pickled vegetables for salads, burgers, sandwiches, cheese plates, or just to eat straight from the jar.

We covered most of this information in our first book, but we've added a few more tips and tricks in here to get you confident and inspired to start pickling at home. Once you understand the craft of pickling, it's really easy and fun. You don't need to make huge batches of pickles to last the whole winter; just start off making a few jars at a time and get your head around the process. Once you get the pickling bug you can conquer the school fete and all your Christmas gifts.

The formula for making pickles is basically always the same. You just have to decide what you're going to pickle; how you're going to prepare the vegetable or fruit; and then which vinegar, sugar and spices you want to use.

WHAT TO PICKLE
Really you can pickle anything. There's a few things we wouldn't recommend — starchy foods such as bananas and potatoes are a bit gross. But as you can see throughout this book, most other vegetables and fruits are delicious pickled.

Our one rule is NEVER pickle anything that is out of season. Vegetables and fruits that are at the height of their season are the most delicious, the freshest and the cheapest. Never buy something imported or frozen to preserve with. It defeats the whole purpose!

For crunchy, tart pickles you need to choose small, freshly picked, firm vegetables that will maintain their texture. This is especially important when pickling fruits. You'll get the best results with very firm unripe fruits — green plums and mangoes, hard pears, etc.

As we're big believers in preserving what is left in the fridge at the end of the week, you can use produce that is starting to deteriorate or soften to make chutneys or relishes, or if you have a couple of wrinkly eggplants (aubergines) or an ageing cauliflower you didn't get to, you can roast them first and then pickle them. Check out the recipe on page 56.

PREPARING YOUR VEGETABLES
Once you've decided what you're going to pickle, there are a few ways to prepare your vegetables to get them ready.

Produce with a high water content, such as cucumbers, zucchini (courgettes), green tomatoes and chokos (chayote), needs to be salted before you start pickling. The salt draws out excess moisture and helps keep your pickles crunchy. It's important to use granulated pure salt, with no iodine or anti-caking agents that can make your brine dark and cloudy.

Sliced pickles, also known as 'bread and butter' pickles, should be salted for a few hours, while whole vegetables such as gherkins or baby zucchini (courgettes) need to be salted overnight. After salting, discard the liquid that has been drawn out of the vegetables. You shouldn't need to rinse the vegetables, but if you've been heavy-handed with the salting, by all means give them a quick rinse and then drain well.

Denser vegetables such as green beans, chillies, celery, beetroot (beets) and carrots can be sliced and put raw straight into the jar. This is the same for most fruits — except quinces, which need to be poached or roasted before they are pickled.

You can also char, smoke or roast vegetables to intensify the flavour. See page 89 for charred jalapeños, and page 128 for roasted pickled fennel. This style of pickling is more like classic antipasti, great for picnics and shared plates.

Some vegetables and fruits might need a quick blanch before you pickle them. Cumquats should be slightly softened in their brine before they go into the jar. Whole beets will need a couple of minutes in boiling water to soften them slightly before pickling. Garlic needs 10 seconds in boiling water to stop it turning blue as it sits in the vinegar brine.

MAKING A BRINE

Your brine is very important. It not only stops bacteria from growing, but is also the difference between an average and a delicious pickle. When you're starting out here's a basic ratio that really works for everything — 4 parts vinegar and 2 parts water to 1 part sugar (4:2:1), plus salt to taste. Once you get a bit more confident with pickling, you'll want to make different brines to match different vegetables and fruits. In this book, we've given you lots of different brine ideas. Start experimenting and find the one you like the most.

It's important you match the vinegar to the produce — so, fruits are great in an apple cider vinegar; white wine vinegar is great for green vegetables and anything you want to maintain the colour and flavour of; red wine vinegar is delicious with beetroot, cherries and red grapes; rice wine vinegar is a good choice for ginger, radish or any Asian style of pickle; and malt vinegar is lovely with onions.

The better quality your vinegar, the better your pickles will be. But you don't need to buy the most expensive vinegar. Instead, try to find mid-range white and red wine vinegars you can buy in larger quantities. Note that vinegar for pickling needs to have an acidity of 5% or higher — this should be indicated on the label. Please avoid straight-up white vinegar. It's so astringent and is really best for cleaning your bathroom!

The sugar you use in your pickles also is important. White or caster (superfine) sugar has no colour or flavour and really is best for pickling vegetables. You want the sugar to soften the acidity of the vinegar, not taste sweet. Don't get stressed about using sugar in pickles. The sugar levels might seem high in a whole recipe, but remember these are condiments, and generally you consume only a tablespoon or two at a sitting, not four jars! Raw sugar is lovely with fruit pickles, and we use brown sugar in our pickled pears and pickled onions. Most other sugars, such as rapadura or coconut sugar, are too strong in flavour and will overpower the pickle.

Remember that sugar alternatives such as honey, stevia and agave can be used as sweeteners, but they're not preserving agents and do not keep bacteria at bay.

To make your brine, put the vinegar, water, sugar and salt (if your vegetables have already been salted or if you are pickling fruits, you can leave the salt out) in a non-reactive saucepan, stirring over low heat to dissolve the sugar. Bring to the boil and let the brine simmer for a few minutes, then turn off the heat.

The flavouring that you add to your pickles is entirely up to you. Remember, it has nothing to do with the preserving process, so feel free to get creative. Whole dried spices such as mustard seeds, fennel seeds, dill seeds and peppercorns are the classic pickle spices, but try different combinations, too. You can add a stick of cinnamon and strip of lemon peel, or a garlic clove and a sprig of rosemary and thyme from the garden. We always recommend a few teaspoons of a few different spices in each jar. Be mindful that the flavours you put in will develop over time; two cloves, a cinnamon stick and a few peppercorns will be delicious, whereas 12 cloves and a tablespoon of peppercorns will be pretty overpowering after a few weeks! Also try to avoid using ground spices, as they make the brine cloudy.

If you have any pickling brine left over, you can store it in a jar in the fridge for up to a month, and use it as a base in salad dressings (see pages 205–206) and for quick pickling (page 162).

PACKING PICKLES INTO JARS
Packing fruit or vegetables perfectly into jars takes practice. You want to get in as much as possible, but without squashing or bruising, or bursting their skins, so you need a firm hand but a gentle touch. Aim to fill the jars to just below the rim, leaving enough room for the vegetables to be completely covered in brine without them touching the lid.

Slowly pour the hot brine over the vegetables, making sure they're completely submerged (anything left uncovered will discolour and deteriorate, and could potentially go mouldy). It's important to get rid of any air bubbles from the jars before sealing them, or the pickles may spoil, because the oxygen in the bubbles enables micro-organisms to thrive. To do this, gently tap each jar on the work surface and slide a clean butter knife or chopstick around the inside of the jar to release any hidden air pockets — you will see bubbles being released from in between the pickles. You may need to add more vegetables or brine afterwards. There needs to be a gap of 5 mm–1.5 cm (¼–⅝ inch) between the brine and the lid — this is called 'headspace', and it allows the vegetables to

expand as they absorb the brine. Keep in mind that smaller and sliced vegetables will absorb less brine than larger ones, so adjust the headspace accordingly.

STORAGE
Wipe the rims of the jars with paper towel or a clean cloth, then put the lids on. If you plan to store your pickles for an extended period, we suggest you heat-process them. Pickles that have been heat-processed and stored correctly — in a cool, dark place — will last for up to 2 years unopened. Make sure you stick to any recommended storage times given in specific recipes. If you don't want to heat-process your pickles, you'll need to store them in the fridge and use them up within a month.

The advantage of heat-processing is that pickles get better over time. Whole pickles need to sit in their jars for at least 6 weeks before use, but will taste even better after 6 months. Sliced pickles are ready after 2 weeks and are best eaten within 6 months, before their texture starts to deteriorate.

Once opened, all pickles should be refrigerated, but will still last for many months in your fridge.

HEAT-PROCESSING
Also called 'water bathing' or 'canning', this process uses heat to stop the growth of bacteria. It generates pressure inside the preserving jar or bottle, which forces out any oxygen, creating an uninhabitable environment for micro-organisms. Treating your preserves in this way has two benefits: it lengthens their shelf life, and it ensures the jars or bottles are sealed correctly. Opinions differ on when heat-processing is necessary, but at Cornersmith we encourage our students to heat-process any cold-packed preserves, pickles and bottled fruit — as well as large batches of chutneys and jams that will be stored for some time.

Get the biggest pan you have, such as a stockpot — the taller, the better — and put it on the stovetop. Lay a folded tea towel in the bottom of the pan, then sit your jars on the tea towel, taking care not to cram them in, and keeping them clear of the sides of the pan. (All these measures are to stop the jars from wobbling around and cracking as the water boils.) Roughly match the water temperature to the temperature of the jars (to help prevent breakages from thermal shock), then pour in enough water to cover the jars, either completely or at least until three-quarters submerged. Bring to the boil over medium heat. The heat-processing times given in the recipes start from boiling point, and will generally be 10–15 minutes for jars or bottles up to 500 ml (17 fl oz/2 cup) capacity, or 20 minutes for larger capacities.

You might have one or two breakages when you're starting out – the worst that can happen is that the remaining jars will swim in pickles for the rest of the processing time. Just keep going, then take the surviving jars out at the end and give them a wipe down. If they all break, you have our permission to have a gin and a lie-down!

Once the heat-processing time is up, the lids should be puffed up and convex. Carefully remove the hot jars from the water. If you've bought some clamps, now is the time to use them, or you can use oven mitts and a thick cloth to protect your hands.

Line your jars up on the benchtop and let them sit overnight. As they cool, a vacuum will form inside each jar and suck down the lid, sealing them securely. In the morning, the lids should be concave: either get down to eye level with the top of the jar to check for the telltale dip in the lid, or lay a pencil across each lid to show the cavity below it.

If you have concerns about the seal of any of your jars (sometimes a couple of jars fail to seal correctly), store them in the fridge and use their contents within a few weeks.

WHICH JARS TO USE

When you're starting out, just use what you've got in the kitchen cupboard. Second-hand jars are fine, as long as there are no cracks or chips in the glass that could harbour micro-organisms or cause the jar to break when heated. Second-hand metal (but not plastic) lids are okay too, if they are in good condition. Make sure there is no rust, and that the white acid-proof coating inside the lids is intact. Also check that the lids aren't misshapen or dented, as both of these can interfere with the seal.

Jars with shoulders or a neck are best for pickling because these help to keep the contents submerged under the brine – you want to avoid vegetables floating to the top and not preserving properly. Also, make sure your jars are tighly packed to keep your pickles under the brine.

If you decide to buy new jars, get good-quality ones made of thick glass – we'd recommend going to a kitchen-supply shop and buying 20 jars and 40 lids. Cheap jars from discount stores often have thin glass, which tends to become brittle and break at high temperatures.

STERILISING JARS AND BOTTLES

To sterilise jars or bottles, give them a wash in hot soapy water and a good rinse, then place upright in a baking dish in a cold oven. Heat the oven to 110°C (225°F) and, once it has reached temperature, leave the jars in the oven for about 10–15 minutes, or until completely dry, then remove them carefully.

For hot packing, pour the hot chutney straight into the hot jars; for cold packing, let the jars cool before adding your pickles or preserves.

To sterilise the lids, place them in a large saucepan of boiling water for 5 minutes, then drain and dry with clean paper towels, or leave them on a wire rack to air dry. Make sure they are completely dry before using.

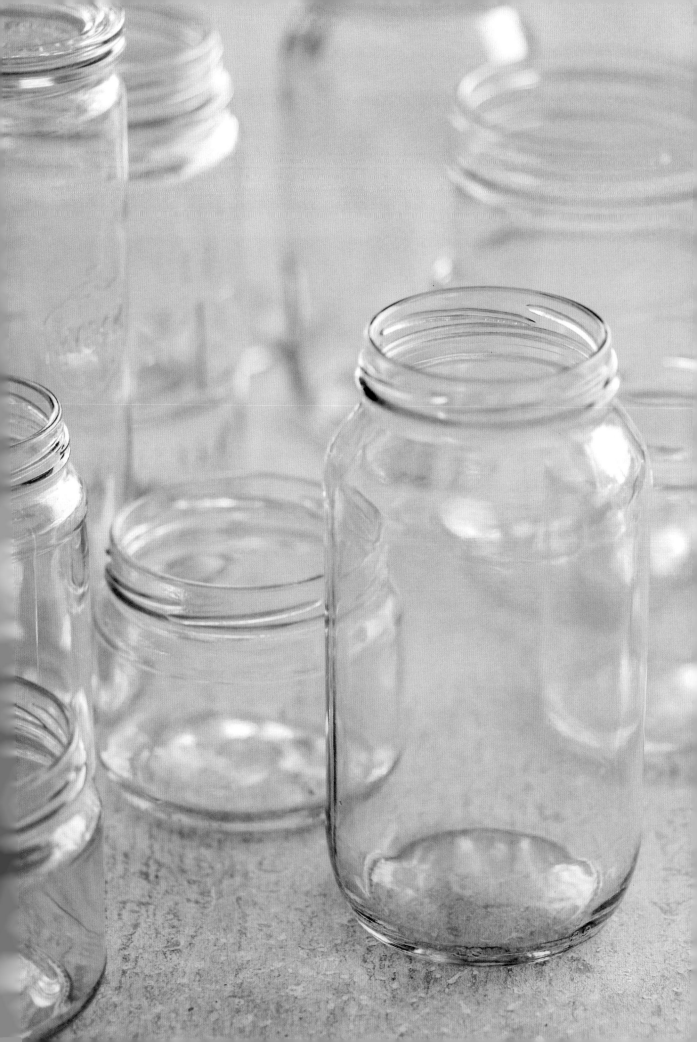

IF YOU REGULARLY MAKE SMALL BATCHES OF CHUTNEY, PICKLES AND SAUCES WITH LEFTOVER FRUIT AND VEGETABLES, YOU'LL NOT ONLY HAVE A PANTRY FULL OF DELICIOUS CONDIMENTS, YOU'LL ALSO REDUCE WHAT GOES INTO YOUR BIN EACH WEEK AND CUT BACK YOUR OVERALL HOUSEHOLD FOOD BUDGET.

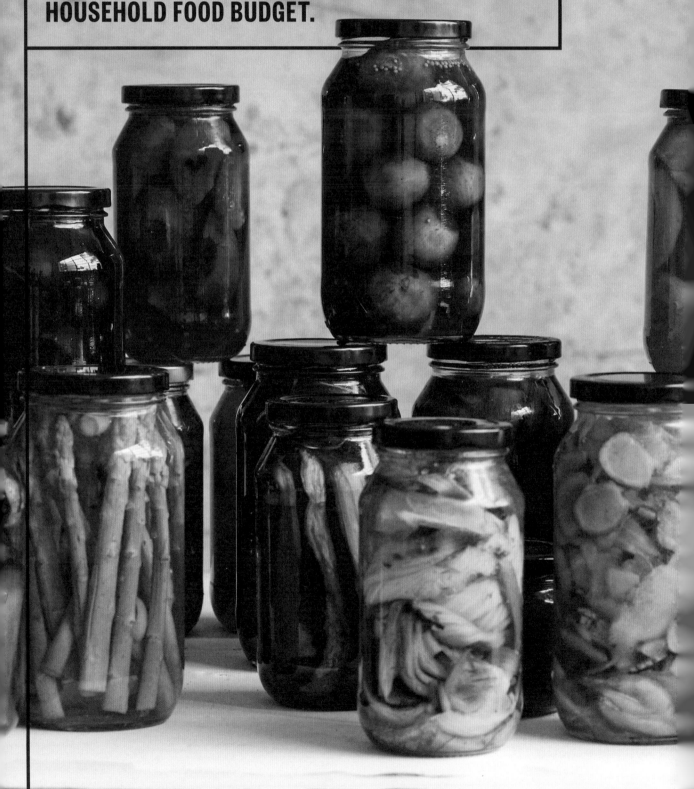

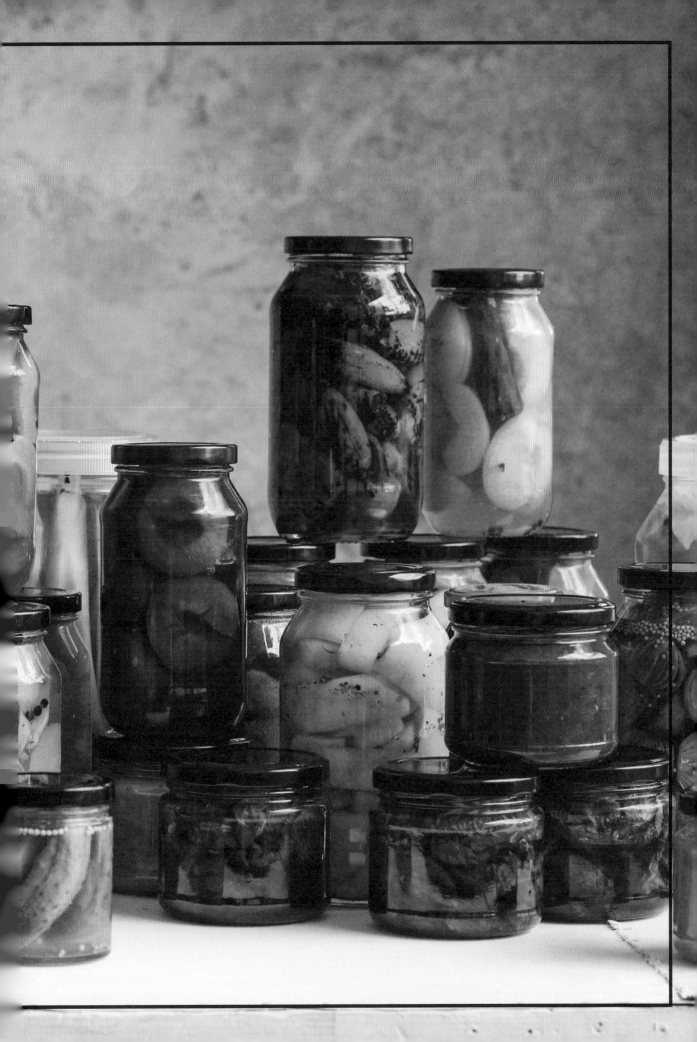

FERMENTING GUIDE

At Cornersmith, we're very lucky to have a resident fermenter, Jaimee Edwards. Jaimee is passionate about the benefits of fermented foods, and here she generously shares her guide to the process, so you can try your hand at fermenting at home.

Fermented foods offer a rich variety of flavours and are beneficial to the health of your gut. They are also very simple to make at home; all you need is seasonal produce, salt and time.

Lacto-fermentation is a very safe method of food preservation. During lacto-fermentation, the lactic acid-producing bacteria (lactobacilli) present on the surface of all fruit and vegetables are encouraged to proliferate in an anaerobic (oxygen-free) environment. Salt is used to inhibit the growth of any harmful bacteria for a few days while the 'good' lactobacilli generate enough lactic acid to preserve the fruit and vegetables. Pure salt should always be used, at a ratio of about 20 g (¾ oz) fine salt to 2 kg (4 lb 8 oz) produce.

Preparing fermented vegetables and fruit is very easy, but once they are packed into their jars you will need to keep an eye on them. Carbon dioxide (one of the natural by-products of fermentation) can build up in your jars, so open your jar every few days to 'burp' your ferment — this will release the built-up carbon dioxide, and prevent brine spilling out of the jar. Just be sure to press down your vegetables afterwards, so that the brine is covering the top by at least 1 cm (½ inch).

Not only does fermenting extend the life of vegetables, it also enhances their nutrient content and digestibility. Even better, consuming fermented foods introduces healthy probiotic bacteria into your gut, which may improve your overall health.

While lacto-fermentation is very safe, as with all food preparation, commonsense and good hygiene practices are needed. Cut away any bruised or perishing parts of your produce; wash and sterilise your jars (see page 212); and keep your hands, benchtops and utensils scrupulously clean.

Once you've packed your produce into jars, fermentation should begin in a few days.

Don't be afraid to try your ferments to see how their flavour is developing. They require a little of your attention — but the reward is that they are foods that really love you back.

Here are some tips on what you need to keep an eye out for.

TIME

The longer you leave your ferment at room temperature, the more its flavour will develop, and the more probiotic bacteria it will contain. Open your jar after a couple of days and see what you think. Your ferment should smell pungent but not foul, and there may be some bubbles. Fermented vegetables have a sour, somewhat yeasty edge to them: think of sourdough bread, strong cheeses and beer.

Depending on the pace of the fermentation and how strong you want the flavour to be, you can leave your jar at room temperature (but out of direct sunlight) for anything from 2 days to 2 weeks before refrigerating — we suggest 2–4 days to start with, but (weather depending) you can ferment for up to 6 weeks.

Trust your palate and instinct when deciding whether your ferment is ready to be moved to the fridge. Your vegetables or fruit will continue to ferment in the fridge, but at a much slower rate, and will keep well for up to 6 months.

TEMPERATURE

In a hot climate, fermentation will be rapid, so during an Australian summer you'll probably need to place your ferments in the refrigerator after 2–3 days. Conversely, in cooler conditions, you may need to wait a week or two for fermentation to take place.

SPILLAGE

As fermentation occurs, you may find that the build-up of carbon dioxide — a natural by-product of the process — forces liquid out of the jar. Just unscrew the lid of your jar and wipe down the rim and sides with paper towel or a clean cloth. If necessary, gently press the vegetables or fruit to re-submerge them in the liquid before replacing the lid.

SAFETY

Once fermentation is underway, the environment in the jar is hostile to harmful bacteria, so relax! Very rarely does anything go wrong. However, if any black mould develops on your ferment, throw the contents of that jar away. If a little white mould is visible on the surface, carefully scoop it off and check underneath: the rest of the ferment may well be fine.

Always trust your instincts, though, especially when you first start fermenting — if something doesn't smell or taste right, discard it.

PRACTICE MAKES PERFECT

When it comes to perfecting the art of fermenting foods, some trial and error is involved, so 'go with the flow', and with time and care you will be well rewarded.

Jaimee Edwards

INDEX

ACKNOWLEDGMENTS

Most importantly we'd like to thank all the Smithies who make
Cornersmith what it is. Your commitment, ideas, enthusiasm and
hard work allow Cornersmith to keep on keeping on. We couldn't
do any of this without you all.

A big thank you to all the Murdoch team — Emma, Hugh and
Katri — for their help in making this project come to life. It's a
beautiful book, which we're very proud of, and we really appreciate
all your support.

To our publisher, Jane Morrow, thank you again for truly
understanding what Cornersmith is all about and why all the little
details are so important to us.

Alan Benson, it's always a pleasure — thank you for your gorgeous
pictures and terrible jokes.

David Morgan, we love you. Thank you for knowing what we like
and for coming up with endless ideas for all the bloody pickles.

Shane Roberts, our incredible vegetable providore and friend, thank
you for filling our kitchens and shops with the best local seasonal
produce and for introducing us to such amazing growers. Without your
generous knowledge and dedication to the seasons we would be lost.

Maddy Dobbins deserves the biggest thank you for being our kitchen
elf, recipe tester, extreme washer-upper, hand model and all round
moral support. Thank you for loving Cornersmith as much as we do.

And, finally, a big thank you to all our customers, students, suppliers,
backyard produce traders and the home cooks who use our cookbooks.
Your constant support and encouragement means everything.

Published in 2017 by Murdoch Books, an imprint of Allen & Unwin

Murdoch Books Australia
83 Alexander Street
Crows Nest NSW 2065
Phone: +61 (0) 2 8425 0100
Fax: +61 (0) 2 9906 2218
murdochbooks.com.au
info@murdochbooks.com.au

Murdoch Books UK
Ormond House
26–27 Boswell Street
London WC1N 3JZ
Phone: +44 (0) 20 8785 5995
murdochbooks.co.uk
info@murdochbooks.co.uk

For Corporate Orders & Custom Publishing, contact our Business Development
Team at salesenquiries@murdochbooks.com.au.

Publisher: Jane Morrow
Editorial Manager: Emma Hutchinson
Designer: Hugh Ford
Editor: Katri Hilden
Photographer: Alan Benson
Stylist: David Morgan
Production: Lou Playfair

A cataloguing-in-publication entry is available from the catalogue of the National
Library of Australia at nla.gov.au.

ISBN 978 1 74336 923 4 Australia
ISBN 978 1 74336 924 1 UK

A catalogue record for this book is available from the British Library.

Colour reproduction by Splitting Image Colour Studio Pty Ltd, Clayton, Victoria
Printed by C & C Offset Printing Co. Ltd., China

IMPORTANT: Those who might be at risk from the effects of salmonella poisoning (the
elderly, pregnant women, young children and those suffering from immune deficiency
diseases) should consult their doctor with any concerns about eating raw eggs.

OVEN GUIDE: You may find cooking times vary depending on the oven you are
using. For fan-forced ovens, as a general rule, set the oven temperature to 20°C
(70°F) lower than indicated in the recipe.

MEASURES GUIDE: We have used 20 ml (4 teaspoon) tablespoon measures. If you
are using a 15 ml (3 teaspoon) tablespoon add an extra teaspoon of the ingredient
for each tablespoon specified.